Management of Medical Emergencies

FOR THE DENTAL TEAM

Management of Medical Emergencies

FOR THE DENTAL TEAM

Martin H. Thornhill MBBS, BDS, PhD
Professor of Oral Medicine,
Department of Oral & Maxillofacial Medicine & Surgery,
University of Sheffield School of Clinical Dentistry,
Claremont Crescent, Sheffield S10 2TA, UK

Michael N. Pemberton MBChB, BDS
Consultant in Oral Medicine
University Dental Hospital of Manchester,
Higher Cambridge Street,
Manchester M15 6FH, UK

Guy J. Atherton BDS, MSc
Orthodontic Practitioner
'The Brace Place', 2 Albert Road,
Crosshills, Keighley BD20 7LE, UK

2005
Published by Stephen Hancocks Limited
27 Bellamy's Court, Abbotshade Road
London, SE16 5RF
www.shancocksltd.com

ISBN 0 954 6145 4 2

Printed and bound by Dennis Barber Limited, Lowestoft, Suffolk

Preface

The aim of this book is to offer a practical guide to dentists and their teams on the management of medical emergencies. We discuss the emergency drugs and equipment that should be available, how to administer drugs and use the equipment, as well as the prevention, diagnosis and initial treatment of acute medical problems that may arise in the dental surgery. It is aimed primarily for readers in the United Kingdom but the principles are universal.

In the first section we deal with the basics as well as the training, equipment, drugs and techniques needed to manage an emergency. In the next section we cover basic life support and management of the collapsed patient. In Section 3, we deal with emergency conditions that usually result in unconsciousness and in the final section with the management of medical emergencies in the conscious patient. For each condition we start with a scenario to give an example of how such an emergency might arise in the dental surgery; we then discuss the causes, signs and symptoms, prevention and management of the condition and, where appropriate, provide additional background information.

Verifiable Continuing Professional Development (CPD)

For dentists and dental care professionals registered with
the UK General Dental Council who are mandated to undertake verifiable
Continuing Professional Development (CPD) a PDF file is available
providing access to a possible 3 hours of CPD.

The PDF file includes 18 questions based on the content of *The Management
of Medical Emergencies*, each with multiple choice answers. Readers can complete and
return the answer sheet, and receive the correct answers and a certificate for
3 hours of verifiable CPD.

The PDF file is available on-line at www.shancocksltd.com or by post from Stephen
Hancocks Limited, 27 Bellamy's Court, Abbotshade Road, London, SE16 5RF
(payment by cheque or credit card – see full payment details on the website)
for £20 including answers and certificate. For further information
please email: shancocks@aol.com

Contents

INTRODUCTION

Dentists and their teams need to be prepared to manage an emergency. As healthcare workers, we have a responsibility to manage any medical problem arising in the dental surgery. The public might also reasonably expect a dentist to be able to offer first line treatment for a medical emergency arising in a public place, until more expert medical assistance arrives. There is therefore an onus on us to be prepared to deal with any such event.

The first aim should be to prevent emergencies from happening. A full understanding of the patient's medical history is of paramount importance in this. Careful treatment planning and patient management in the full knowledge of the medical history will prevent the majority of emergencies from occurring. Should an emergency occur, however, the main aim must be to keep the patient alive until they can be transferred to more expert medical care for definitive treatment - usually in the accident and emergency department of the nearest hospital. Since the speed with which a patient receives expert care can be critical in determining the chances of survival, the first priority must be to alert the emergency services. The next priority is to prevent, as far as possible, any deterioration in the patient's condition before assistance arrives. Bearing this in mind, it seems reasonable to expect a dentist to diagnose the main acute life threatening events such as myocardial infarction, cardiac arrest and anaphylaxis. They and their team should also have the skills to assess the patient, maintain the patency of the airway, carry out basic life support, including administration of positive pressure air or oxygen and, if trained, carry out defibrillation and deliver emergency drugs. Preparation to deal with such events effectively and with a minimum of stress requires regular training and the availability of appropriate emergency equipment and drugs. It is essential that all members of the dental team, including nurses and reception staff, are involved in medical emergency training.

Fainting occurs quite often in dental practice but fortunately other medical emergencies are uncommon. A recent survey found that, apart from faints, on average a medical emergency event occurred once every $3\frac{1}{2}$ to $4\frac{1}{2}$ years of practice in Great Britain and an event in which cardiopulmonary resuscitation (CPR) was required occurred once every 200 to 250 years. However, the stress felt by many patients when attending the dental surgery, and the nature of dental treatment mean that the risk of an emergency occurring in a dental surgery is higher than in most other settings. If a medical emergency occurs, it is likely to be unexpected and alarming, not just for the patient, but for all members of the team and other patients, and may even be life threatening to your patient.

Medical emergencies in children are even more rare. Because of their rarity, the guidelines for management of medical emergencies given here apply only to adults and would need to be modified for use in young children. In general the principles for treating children are the same as for adults. However, drug dosages need to be adjusted and anatomical and physiological differences may necessitate modification of management procedures.

Even though we have provided guidelines for the use of emergency drugs and equipment in the dental surgery, emergency management protocols are under constant review and it is important to keep abreast of any changes that occur.

PREVENTION AND PREPARATION

Many factors contribute to preventing medical emergencies from occurring and many are common sense. They include the ambience of the practice, the training and attitude of staff and your knowledge of the patient's medical history.

THE PRACTICE

Comfortable practice surroundings and a friendly atmosphere are of benefit not only in promoting the good reputation of the practice but also help allay the fears of more anxious patients and generate a feeling of confidence and well being. On a more practical level, it is important that you have easy access to all parts of the surgery premises used by patients, including the lavatory, which it should be possible to unlock from the outside. Getting an acutely ill patient lying flat is a major priority and it should be possible to do this with relative ease in all parts of the surgery.

THE TEAM

The professionalism and attitude of the dental team plays an important part in allaying patients' fears and preventing stressful situations from arising that could potentially result in a medical emergency. Informed and observant staff may also identify emergency situations at an early stage so that preventive action can be taken.

On a practical level, it is essential that all team members know where the emergency drugs and equipment are kept and are properly trained and prepared to deal with an emergency, including a collapsed patient. Resuscitation skills should be practised regularly as a team in simulated emergencies. Training should take place in the dental surgery and in the waiting area to familiarise all team members with dealing with emergencies in different locations and ensure there is space to deploy equipment properly. Ideally, an accredited instructor should give training and each person who undergoes training should have his or her proficiency tested and certified.

In many areas there are schemes in operation, often run by the local post-graduate dean's office, which provide 'hands on' CPR training for the dental team in their own dental practice; some areas also provide training in the management of other types of medical emergency. In rehearsing staff for dealing with an emergency, it is important to ensure that each member of staff knows what is expected of them, who will telephone for assistance and what they should say, who will get the emergency equipment and who will take charge. A notice next to the telephone with concise instructions, including the address details of the surgery, can be helpful in ensuring the right details are given, particularly when new or temporary staff may be managing the reception.

MEDICAL HISTORY

Obtaining a medical history is an essential step in evaluating a patient and how their dental treatment should be managed. A substantial and increasing number of patients attending the dental surgery have medical conditions or are taking medication which may influence their dental management. In view of this, the medical history should be obtained from every patient and updated at every recall. It should include enquiries about:

- current medication
- current treatment by doctor or hospital specialist or clinic
- allergies to medicines, substances (e.g. metals or latex) or foods
- cardiovascular disease or increased blood pressure
- a history of rheumatic fever
- the nature of any heart surgery
- respiratory disease (including asthma or bronchitis)
- endocrine disorders (e.g. diabetes)
- epilepsy
- excessive bleeding, especially after extractions
- any other serious illnesses
- if the patient may be pregnant.

The patient's medical history will often suggest the type of medical problem to be anticipated; diabetics who use insulin are at most risk of hypoglycaemia, especially if treated just before they are due to eat a meal. Patients with angina have ischaemic heart disease and will be more likely to suffer a myocardial infarct. Forearmed with such knowledge, it may be possible to take steps to reduce the likelihood of any problems arising during treatment.

Printed medical history forms can be used but it is advisable to seek verbal confirmation from the patient of what has been written. A suggested medical history form is shown in *Figure 1.1*; other designs of medical history form are available from various sources including the British Dental Association (BDA)[1] and Admor Ltd[2]. Any points arising from enquiries about the medical history should be investigated further. Look up any drugs you are not familiar with in the British National Formulary, Merck Manual or other such source. If there is anything about which you or the patient are not clear, it is worth looking it up in a medical textbook such as Scully and Cawsons' *Medical Problems in Dentistry*[3]; where you feel additional clarification would be useful, you should contact the patient's medical practitioner or hospital specialist.

Figure 1.1. A medical history form

CONFIDENTIAL MEDICAL HISTORY FORM

To obtain the best and safest treatment your dentist needs to know of any medical problems which may affect your treatment.

It would also help if you bring any **medicines** you are taking and the **name and address of your doctor**.

No medical problem or infection will exclude you from essential treatment.

This form is to be completed by the patient, parent or guardian.

NAME: last   first   other

ADDRESS

TELEPHONE: home   work   DATE OF BIRTH

	NO	YES	DETAILS
DO YOU:			
1 Attend or receive treatment from a doctor, hospital, or clinic?			
2 Take any medicines or drugs (injections, tablets, creams etc)?			
3 Take or have you taken any steroids in the last 2 years?			
4 Have an allergy to any medicines, foods or materials?			
5 Suffer from hay fever, asthma, eczema or any other allergy?			
6 Have a heart problem, murmur, angina, high blood pressure?			
7 Suffer from bronchitis, shortness of breath or other chest condition?			
8 Have diabetes?			
9 Have fainting attacks, giddiness, blackouts or epilepsy?			
HAVE YOU:			
10 Ever had Rheumatic Fever or Chorea (St Vitus' Dance)?			
11 Ever had jaundice, liver disease or hepatitis?			
12 Had cause to think you are infected with TB, hepatitis or HIV?			
13 Had a bad reaction to a local or general anaesthetic?			
14 Bled excessively following a tooth extraction, surgery or injury?			
15 Had any serious illnesses, disabilities, or operations?			
DO YOU:			
16 Have a pacemaker, or have you had any form of heart surgery?			
17 Do you have any disease, condition or problem not listed above that you think your doctor/dentist should know about?			
HOW MUCH:			
18 Do you smoke per day?			
19 Alcohol do you drink per day / week?			
WOMEN ONLY:			
20 Are you pregnant or breast feeding?			

Doctor's name and address:..

.... Doctor's Tel No........................

Signature:.................................... Checked by

Date:.................................... Date

EMERGENCY EQUIPMENT

Various authorities give guidelines on the emergency equipment that should be available in a dental surgery. Our list is similar to such recommendations.

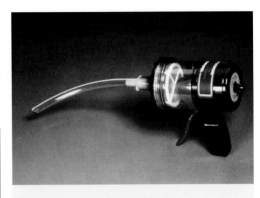

Figure 1.2: Hand held aspirator

SUGGESTED EMERGENCY EQUIPMENT FOR THE DENTAL SURGERY

- Efficient, portable aspirator (to clear the airway)
- Oxygen supply and mask, capable of delivering 10L/min;
- Airway adjuncts
- A ventilation mask (e.g. Laerdal® Pocket Mask)
- A selection of oropharyngeal (Guedal) airways (sizes 2, 3 and 4 for respectively small, medium and large adults)
- A bag and valve manual ventilator (e.g. AMBU® bag) - the best device for delivering positive pressure air or oxygen
- Selection of disposable syringes (1, 2, 5 and 10 mL*) and needles (19 gauge (white hub), 21 gauge (green), 23 gauge (blue) and 25 gauge (orange))
- Butterfly needles or intravenous (i/v) cannulae (19 or 21 gauge)
- A tourniquet

Optional:

- If available, an RA machine or Entonox (for analgesia in the management of myocardial infarction)
- An automatic external defibrillator (AED)

*50ml syringe may be needed if you keep 50ml ampoules of 20% glucose solution for injection in your emergency drug kit.

AIRWAY ADJUNCTS

VENTILATION MASK (Pocket Mask)

These masks[6,8,9] are designed to avoid the necessity of actual mouth-to-mouth contact during expired air ventilation. You can attach a one-way valve, which directs the patient's exhaled air away from you. The mask is made of clear plastic so that you can see if the patient has vomited or is bleeding. In addition, there is a nozzle that allows a source of oxygen to be attached to supplement your expired air and enrich it with oxygen. These ventilation masks can also be used, without the one-way valve, in conjunction with a bag and valve manual ventilator, such as an Ambu Bag®[7], which has it own one-way valve.

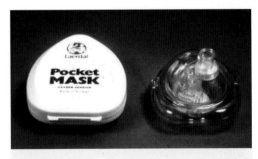

Figure 1.3. Pocket mask with non-return valve attached

The mask is used by pressing it tightly against the skin of the face around the mouth and nose while at the same time pulling the mandible forward to maintain patency of the airway (*Figure 1.4*). If there is difficulty in maintaining patency of the airway, then an oropharyngeal (Guedal) airway may help.

PORTABLE ASPIRATOR

Even if your surgery uses portable aspirators, which can be wheeled around the surgery and to all parts of the practice premises, a small, portable, hand-held aspirator, powered by a hand or foot pump is advisable in addition. If you have no other form of portable suction, one of these is essential. It is vital, in management of a collapsed patient, that the airway is cleared of blood and vomit and maintained at all times. Hand or foot-pump powered aspirators are available from various sources (e.g. Vitalograph®[4]; Emergency Medical Services Res-Q-Vac®[5]; Laerdal V-Vac®[6] or Ambu Res-Cue Pump®[7])

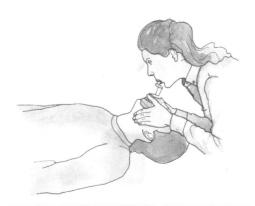

Figure 1.4. Pocket mask being used with a non-return valve

OROPHARYNGEAL (GUEDAL) AIRWAYS

Oropharyngeal airways are adjuncts which can be used to improve the patency of the airway and allow more efficient artificial ventilation to be carried out if, for example, the patient's lips are closed; they are also helpful in overcoming the backward displacement of the tongue in an unconscious individual. They do not protrude from the face and so can be used with a ventilation mask.

They consist of a curved plastic tube with a flange at the oral end and have a flattened shape to ensure they fit neatly between the tongue and the hard palate. If the airway used is too long, it may induce laryngospasm or vomiting in a patient who is not deeply unconscious. They are available in various sizes; sizes 2, 3 and 4 are suitable for adults. To estimate the correct size of airway for a particular

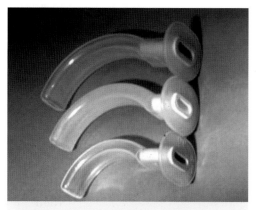

Figure 1.5. Oropharyngeal airways

patient select an airway with a length corresponding to the distance from the angle of the patient's mouth to the tragus at the front of the ear.

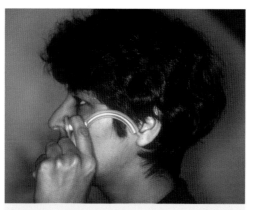

Figure 1.6. Finding the correct size oropharyngeal airway

An oropharyngeal airway is inserted upside down initially and rotated through 180° as it passes back over the tongue so that the tip of the airway eventually faces down toward the larynx.

BAG AND VALVE MANUAL VENTILATORS

The use of a bag and valve manual ventilator in conjunction with the ventilation mask obviates any risk to the rescuer from contact with the victim and allows greater volumes of air to be

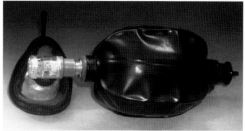

Figure 1.7. Bag and valve manual ventilator

delivered with a greater oxygen concentration than expired air. It is difficult for one person to squeeze the bag at the same time as maintaining the mask seal and airway. Thus, if possible, two people should be involved; one person to maintain the mask seal and keep the airway patent, while the other pumps the bag to give positive pressure ventilation

(Figure 1.8). Connecting an oxygen supply to the bag increases the concentration of oxygen delivered still further. The use of oxygen with flow rates of 8-12L/min will allow air with a 80-95% concentration of oxygen to be delivered.

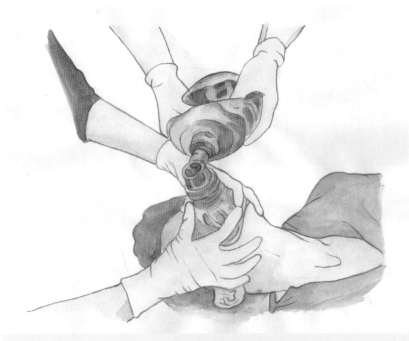

Figure 1.8. Two person operation of ventilation bag/mask

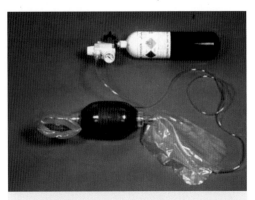

Figure 1.9. Bag and valve manual ventilator with oxygen supply and reservoir bag attached

OXYGEN SUPPLY

A supply of oxygen is essential for increasing the oxygen concentration being delivered to the patient's lungs in cases of hypoxia (respiratory impairment) or anoxia (respiratory arrest). Both ventilation masks and manual ventilators have nozzles that allow oxygen to be attached. An oxygen cylinder that can deliver up to 10 litres per minute should be used. The size of oxygen cylinder you require is determined by how long you might need to use oxygen before assistance arrives. You may consider having a larger cylinder if you work in a rural area or where traffic congestion may result in a longer journey time for an ambulance. A 'D' size cylinder holds 340 litres and will give 10L/min for 34 minutes whereas an 'E' size cylinder holds 680 litres and will last approximately 68 minutes. In the UK, oxygen cylinders can be obtained from Blackwells Anaesthetic Supplies Ltd.[10], BOC Gases[11], Linde Gas UK Ltd. [12].

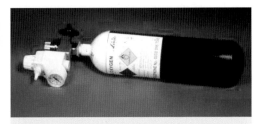

Figure 1.10. Oxygen cylinder

OXYGEN DELIVERY MASK

A loose fitting oxygen delivery mask is used to supplement the oxygen concentration being delivered to a patient who is breathing but is not doing so effectively and is therefore hypoxic. An oxygen flow rate of 10L/min should be used. This type of mask has holes in it to ensure ambient air, including CO_2, is also entrained. The entrained CO_2 stimulates the breathing centre of the brain and helps maintain the patient's drive to breathe.

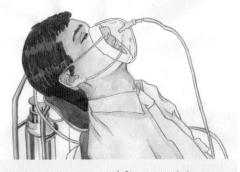

Figure 1.11. Oxygen delivery mask in use

TOURNIQUET

This is used to engorge the veins with blood to make them easier to identify for venepuncture. These can be obtained from many sources (e.g. Blackwells[10]), however, if nothing else is available, a rubber examination glove can be stretched and tied round the arm.

SYRINGES, NEEDLES, BUTTERFLIES, INTRAVENOUS CANNULAE

Use a syringe appropriate to the volume of the drug you are going to give: a 1mL syringe is far more appropriate for giving 1mL of a drug than would be a 20mL syringe. Generally 25 gauge needles, usually with an orange hub, are used for subcutaneous injections, 23 gauge (blue hub) needles are used for intramuscular injections and 21 gauge (green) needles are used for intravenous (i/v) injections. For more viscous solutions (e.g. 20% glucose solution), a wider, 19 gauge (white) needle will be necessary. If i/v drugs need to be given repeatedly, in a large volume or the patient is hard to keep still during injection, a butterfly or i/v cannula will make administration easier. However, this is only the case if you are trained and confident in their use.

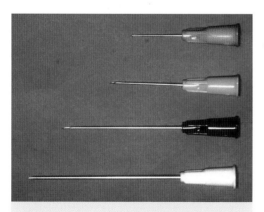

Figure 1.12. Commonly used needle sizes

RELATIVE ANALGESIA EQUIPMENT OR ENTONOX

Nitrous oxide is an effective means of reducing pain and anxiety in a patient suffering from myocardial infarct. Relative analgesia equipment is usually able to deliver an appropriate mix of 50% nitrous oxide and 50% oxygen for this purpose.

For practices without RA equipment, an Entonox cylinder, delivery system and mask is an alternative.

AUTOMATIC EXTERNAL DEFIBRILLATOR

In management of cardiac arrest, the sooner the patient is defibrillated the better the prognosis for survival. In view of this, automatic external defibrillators (AEDs) have been developed and are widely available on aircraft, in public buildings and on public service vehicles such as police cars and fire engines. They are

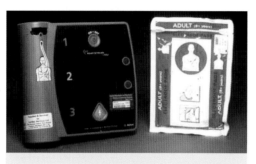

Figure 1.13. Automatic External Defibrillator (AED) with disposable electrode pads

simple to use and can be successfully operated by non-medical personnel after minimal training. After placing the chest pads, the AED will lead you through the entire process of defibrillation using voice prompts and visual messages on a screen. They will automatically analyse the heart's rhythm and determine whether a shock is required or not and provide the correct sequence of shocks with minimal input from you. Many existing AEDs are monophasic defibrillators and provide a sequence of shocks at 200, 200 and 360 joules. However, most of the newer devices are biphasic and deliver lower energy shocks. The cost of AEDs has reduced significantly and a growing number of dental practices now have these devices. Currently an AED costs in the region of £2,000. However, prices are falling and there is a case to be made for dental surgeries having one, especially in isolated communities some distance from an ambulance service. They are available from a number of companies including Laerdal[6], Life Tec Medical Ltd[13], Medtronic[14], and Philips Medical Systems[15]. They are also available through www.aed4u.com.

EMERGENCY DRUGS

The Poswillo Report, published in 1990, made recommendations about the emergency drugs and equipment that should be available in dental practices in the UK. Some felt these recommendations were excessive for the majority of practices that did not carry out general anaesthesia (GA). Now that GA is no longer carried out in general dental practice, the current consensus is to stock fewer drugs. In England, Wales and Northern Ireland the emergency drugs listed in the introductory section of the British National Formulary (BNF), entitled *Medical Emergencies in Dental Practice* provides a suitable list. This lists 12 emergency drugs, outlined in *Table 1*, that should be available to assist with first line treatment of a medical emergency arising in a dental surgery. It does not include drugs for advanced cardiac life support. The BNF is updated every six months and its recommendations do change from time to time.

a much more streamlined list of five 'essential drugs': oxygen; adrenaline; glucagon; a salbutamol inhaler and glyceryl trinitrate (GTN) spray. However, the BNF's list is probably the most comprehensive and provides a good basis for dealing with most emergencies that are likely to arise in the dental surgery; it includes all the drugs described in this book.

Commercial emergency 'kits', which contain all the necessary drugs and equipment are available (e.g. Blackwells[10] produce one). Whether you choose a commercial emergency drug kit or create your own, it is essential to be familiar with all the emergency drugs and equipment you possess, know how to use them and replace the drugs before they pass their 'use by' date. The commercial kits often provide a notification system to replace drugs that are soon to go out of date; if you have created your own drug kit, you should devise a system to ensure that they are replaced before this happens. A good method is to make a note in the practice appointment book when a drug needs to be replaced. Some computer practice management systems have the facility to provide reminders.

Practitioners who carry out intravenous sedation should do so only after appropriate training and must ensure that they have equipment necessary to deal with any emergency situation arising from its use and carry appropriate additional drugs, such as flumazenil, the benzodiazepine antagonist. We have not specifically discussed problems arising from the use of intravenous sedation or general anaesthesia as it falls beyond the scope of this book.

Table 1. Emergency drugs

EMERGENCY DRUGS RECOMMENDED BY THE BRITISH NATIONAL FORMULARY.

The suggested minimum quantities to be kept in the emergency kit are shown in brackets.

- Epinephrine (adrenaline) injection 1:1000, 1mg/mL, 1mL ampoules (3-4)

- Aspirin dispersible tablets 300mg

- Chlorphenamine (Chlorpheniramine) injection, 10mg/mL, 1mL ampoules (2-3)

- Diazepam injection, 5mg/mL, 2mL ampoules (2)

- Glucagon injection, 1 unit (1mg) vials (with solvent) (1)

- Glucose powder or syrup (e.g. Hypostop®)

- Glucose 20% intravenous infusion, 200mg/mL, 50ml ampoules (1)

- Glyceryl trinitrate spray or tablets (1 spray)

- Hydrocortisone sodium succinate 100mg (with 2mL ampoule of water) for injection. (2)

- Oxygen (1 x 'E' size cylinder)

- Salbutamol aerosol inhaler, 100 micrograms/metered dose (1)

- Salbutamol injection 500 micrograms/mL; 1mL ampoules (1)

Other authorities and organisations[16-21] have made recommendations for emergency drugs and equipment which should be available in a dental practice. The Scottish Office[16], for example, recommends

ADMINISTERING EMERGENCY DRUGS

For a drug to be effective in an emergency, it must be got into the patient by a means that will ensure rapid absorption and therapeutic effect. The main routes of drug administration are:

- **By mouth**

    (a) topically across the oral mucosa. Glyceryl trinitrate placed under the

tongue is absorbed rapidly across the mucosa of the floor of the mouth and is used in the treatment of angina.

(b) *systemically.* If a hypoglycaemic diabetic patient is conscious, a glucose preparation, such as glucose powder dissolved in water or Hypostop®, a glucose rich syrup designed to be absorbed across the mucosa, can be administered. For other emergency drugs the rate of absorption of the drug is usually too slow by the oral route.

• **By inhalation** - this affords rapid absorption of some drugs. It is especially effective if the target organ is the lungs, hence an inhaler or nebuliser is the best way of administering salbutamol in the treatment of asthma. This route is rapid in effect and minimises systemic side effects.

• **By rectum** – this is only appropriate for giving diazepam in status epilepticus.

• **By injection.** There are three routes:
  • intravenous (i/v)
  • intramuscular (i/m)
  • subcutaneous (s/c).

DRUG DELIVERY TECHNIQUES
ADMINISTERING DRUGS BY INJECTION
INTRAVENOUS INJECTION
Intravenous (i/v) injection affords the most rapid distribution of a drug. Most dentists have had some experience in gaining i/v access but this will usually have been on fit young patients with good veins and may have been some time ago. In a medical emergency, it is unlikely to be as straightforward; first because you will be under pressure and second because the patient is likely to be shocked, the peripheral vasculature may be shut down. The difficulty of gaining i/v access in emergencies is now widely recognised and guidelines for emergency drug use by dentists increasingly recommend administration by other routes. Our advice is that if you feel competent to get i/v access then do so but don't waste valuable time on repeated attempts. If you are not successful at first - try other routes for

administering emergency drugs.

The antecubital fossa is usually the best site to gain i/v access. Secure a tourniquet above the patient's elbow and make sure it is tight enough to inhibit venous return; if the patient is conscious, ask them to clench and unclench their fist repeatedly. Slapping the injection site with your forefinger and middle finger may also help engorge the veins. Approach the vein with the needle as near parallel with the vein as possible, with the bevel of the needle uppermost. Pierce the skin and enter the vein; entering at the junction of two veins is often easier. Once in the vein, the tourniquet should be released before injecting the drug slowly.

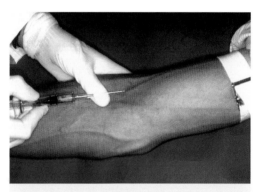

Figure 1.14. Inserting a needle into a vein in the ante-cubital fossa

Drugs which can be administered by i/v injection:

• hydrocortisone - in acute steroid insufficiency and as an adjunct in anaphylaxis

• chlorphenamine (chlorpheniramine) - in acute allergic reactions and as an adjunct in anaphylaxis

• diazepam - in status epilepticus (where there are repeated bouts of grand mal fitting)

• glucose solution - in an unconscious hypoglycaemic patient

• glucagon - in an unconscious hypoglycaemic patient.

Many emergency drugs are supplied in clear glass vials. Simply break open the vial at the neck and draw the liquid into

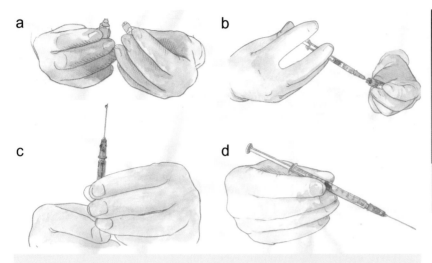

Figure 1.15. Drawing up a drug from a vial; (a) break open vial, (b) draw up drug into syringe using a needle, (c) expel air from the syringe, (d) ready to inject

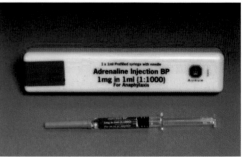

Figure 1.17. Aurum pre-loaded epinephrine (adrenaline) syringe

the syringe via a needle. Expel any air from the syringe before injecting (*Figure 1.15*).

As an aid to rapid administration, a number of emergency drugs are now available for immediate use. One such system is the 'Min-i-jet' system[22] (*Figure 1.16*). This consists of a glass vial that forms the plunger of the syringe. To prepare the drug for injection, remove the yellow protective caps and insert the glass vial into the plastic syringe prior to injection. Another pre-loaded syringe system is produced by Aurum[23] (*Figure 1.17*).

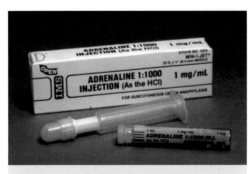

Figure 1.16. Mini-jet pre-loaded epinephrine (adrenaline) syringe system

Hydrocortisone is not stable for any length of time in a liquid form and is supplied as a powder, which you dissolve in sterile water (supplied) to make the preparation for injection (*Figure 1.18*). In this case,

break open the vial of sterile water (2mL) and draw it up into the syringe with a needle. Remove the cover from the vial of powder, insert the needle of the syringe containing the sterile water through the rubber bung and inject the water into the vial (*Figure 1.19*). Agitate until the powder is completely dissolved and draw the liquid back into the syringe. Expel any air before injecting it.

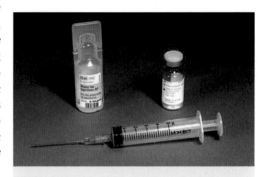

Figure 1.18. Hydrocortisone comes as a vial of water and a vial of powder that need to be mixed

INTRAMUSCULAR INJECTION
Many drugs can be given i/m, although they are not disseminated as rapidly as drugs given i/v, eventual blood levels can be comparable with those achieved by i/v bolus injection. I/m injections can be administered at four sites:

• the upper arm (deltoid muscle)(*Figure 1.20*)

• the upper outer quadrant of the buttock (gluteus medius muscle) (*Figure 1.21*)

• the thigh (vastus lateralis muscle) (*Figure 1.22*)

• the muscle mass of the tongue –

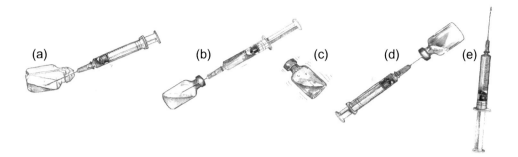

Figure 1.19. Five stages of preparing hydrocortisone for injection. (a) draw up sterile water, (b) inject water into vial of hydrocortisone powder, (c) shake to mix, (d) draw up hydrocortisone solution (e) expel air from syringe

familiar territory for dentists (*Figure 1.23*).

The safest site is the thigh. Use a 23 gauge (blue) needle. Even in the most wasted individual there is sufficient muscle bulk, absorption will be relatively rapid and there is minimal chance of damaging any other structure. In an emergency this site is also accessible through clothing. You should aim for the middle of the antero-lateral aspect of the thigh, midway between the top of the leg and the knee. The upper arm and upper outer quadrant of the buttock are less accessible and involve the risk of damage to the radial nerve in the arm and sciatic nerve in the buttock should the injections be misplaced.

Having loaded the syringe with the drug you wish to give, disinfect the skin with some form of alcohol wipe. Stretch the skin with one hand and insert the needle with a stabbing action through the skin, at 90° to the surface, into the muscle. Before injecting aspirate to check that you are not in a blood vessel. If you aspirate blood, withdraw the needle slightly and try again. When you no longer aspirate blood, inject the solution slowly then withdraw the needle quickly, pressing on the

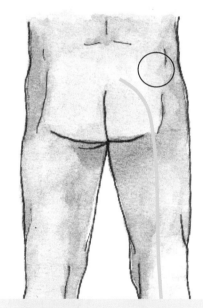

Figure 1.21. I/m injection site (red circle) in upper outer quadrant of buttock (to avoid route of sciatic nerve shown in yellow)

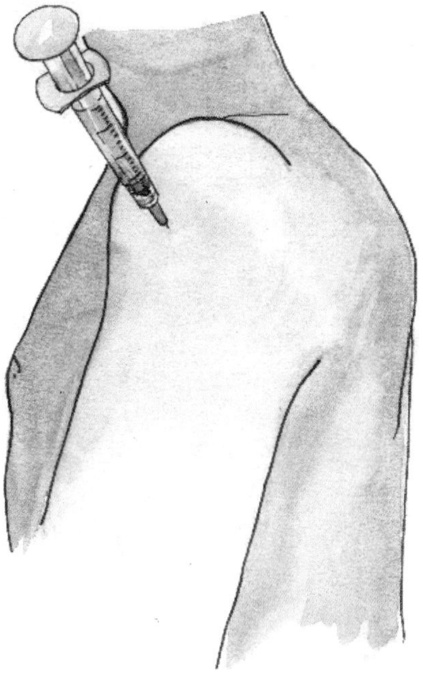

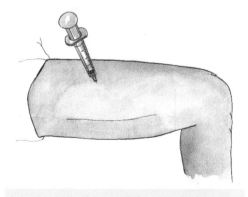

Figure 1.20. I/m injection into arm

Figure 1.22. I/m injection into thigh

injection site with a gauze swab and massage gently.

The tongue has a smaller muscle bulk than muscles at other sites but is readily accessible to a dentist. In an emergency, if other sites are inaccessible, it may accommodate injection of a small amount

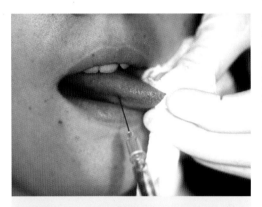

Figure 1.23. I/m injection into the tongue

of fluid, up to 1mL.
Drugs that can be given by i/m injection:

- epinephrine (adrenaline) - in anaphylaxis

- hydrocortisone - in acute steroid insufficiency and as an adjunct in anaphylaxis

- glucagon - in an unconscious hypoglycaemic patient

- chlorphenamine (chlorpheniramine) - in acute allergic reactions and as an adjunct in anaphylaxis.

SUBCUTANEOUS INJECTION
In an emergency, subcutaneous injection is always a second choice. Absorption of a drug from this site is slower and less predictable than from muscle and is only suitable for small volumes (1mL or less). Nevertheless should you be unable to give a drug by any other means, then this route can be used. The aim is to deposit the drug in the loose connective tissue under the skin. The best sites for injection are where there is subcutaneous fat such as:

- the outer upper arm

- the abdomen below the ribs

- anterior thighs.

The best site is the abdomen, as even the thinnest individual has some fat in this region. Use a 25 gauge orange needle to deliver small volumes (up to 1mL). Load the syringe and have the needle in place. If a suitable disinfecting agent is at hand, wipe it over the skin, then pinch about two inches of flesh between forefinger and thumb. Insert the needle through the skin at an angle of 45° with a short stabbing action. Aspirate to ensure that you are not in a blood vessel before injecting the drug slowly. Withdraw the needle quickly and place a disinfectant or gauze swab over the injection site and massage it lightly.

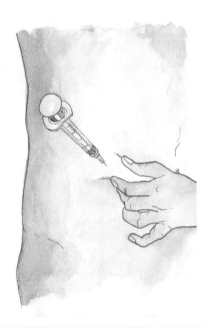

Figure 1.24. Subcutaneous injection into the abdominal skin

Drugs that can be given by s/c injection:

- epinephrine (adrenaline) in treatment of anaphylaxis (first choice route: i/m)

- glucagon in hypoglycaemia (first choice route: i/m)

- salbutamol in asthma (first choice route: inhalation).

ADMINISTERING DRUGS
BY INHALATION
Aerosol preparations, such as salbutamol inhalers, are usually carried by asthmatics and those with chronic obstructive

pulmonary disease (COPD); these patients should be proficient in the use of them. They come in several forms: the most common are the pressurised (aerosol) inhalers which require the patient to activate the inhaler while breathing in and holding their breath for ten seconds afterwards. For those unable to use such inhalers, breath activated aerosol inhalers, dry powder inhalers and spacing devices are available – make sure that the patient has any specialised inhalers with them when they attend for treatment.

Patients suffering an acute asthmatic attack can find it difficult to coordinate a deep inspiration with triggering of the inhaler. Indeed, they may be unable to take a deep breath at all; as a result the jet from the inhaler may deposit at the back of the throat rather than entering the lungs. In these cases a large volume spacer device placed between the inhaler and the mouth may help.

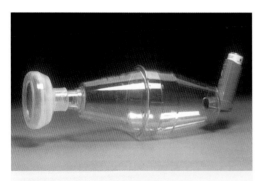

Figure 1.25. Inhaler with spacer

The spacer reduces the velocity of the drug and mixes it more effectively with

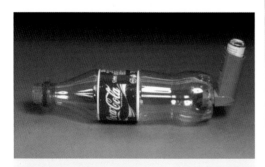

Figure 1.26. Soft drinks bottle used as spacer for inhaler

any inspired air. In an emergency, if a proper spacer is not available, one can be fashioned from a large disposable cup or 500ml soft drink bottle.

More effective still is to nebulise the drug and deliver it along with oxygen via a mask.

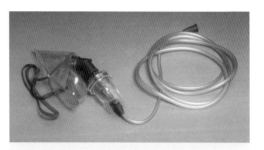

Figure 1.27. Oxygen delivery mask with a nebuliser attachment

Oxygen delivery masks with an attached nebuliser chamber can be purchased very cheaply. They can be used as an oxygen delivery mask with or without using the nebuliser facility. When used as a nebuliser, the drug (e.g. a nebule of salbutamol (1mg/mL, 2.5mls i.e. 2.5mg)) is emptied into the nebuliser chamber and the oxygen turned on. The oxygen and nebulised drug are delivered very effectively into the patient's lungs, via the mask, even when their breaths are very shallow or laboured.

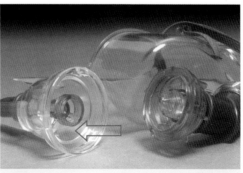

Figure 1.28 Close up of open nebuliser chamber (arrow shows where salbutamol, or other drug for delivery, is placed)

SUBLINGUAL ADMINISTRATION

Patients who require glyceryl trinitrate (GTN) for relief of angina usually carry a sublingual spray with them and should be

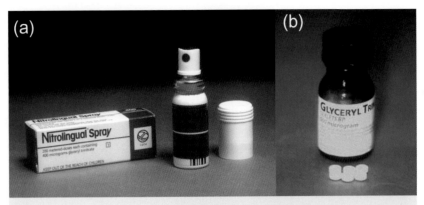

Figure 1.29. Sublingual glyceryl trinitrate (a) spray and (b) tablets

practised in its use (*Figure 1.29*). If there is any doubt, ask the patient to open his or her mouth and lift the tongue to the roof of the mouth, then spray the floor of the mouth with two squirts of the GTN spray.

PER RECTAL ADMINISTRATION
OF DRUGS
Absorption across the rectal mucosa is good and a number of drugs can be given by this route. However, the only emergency situation in a dental surgery where it may be reasonable to consider this route is to give diazepam to a patient having repeated epileptic seizures (status epilepticus). Intravenous administration is preferable but can be difficult in a patient having seizures.

With the patient in the recovery position, expose the buttocks. Break off the seal of the rectal diazepam applicator, gently insert the applicator tubing into the rectum and press the plastic vial to administer the drug.

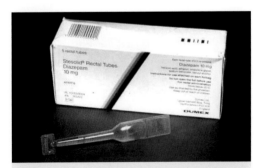

Figure 1.30. Diazepam rectal tube for
PR delivery

2

INTRODUCTION

In this section we discuss the management of the collapsed patient. We start by covering the principles of basic life support (BLS). We then discuss the chain of survival for cardiac arrest and the importance of defibrillation. In particular we discuss the increasing use of automatic external defibrillators (AEDs) and the role of advanced life support training in improving the outcome of cardiac arrest. We then cover the difficult diagnostic problem of the patient who collapses in the dental surgery where the cause is not known. In Section 3 we discuss in more detail the management of the different individual causes of collapse.

BASIC LIFE SUPPORT (BLS)

The procedures described in this section are based on the guidelines of the Resuscitation Council (UK). These guidelines are updated periodically and can be checked on the Resuscitation Council's web site[24].

Without adequate ventilation of the lungs to oxygenate the blood and without an adequate circulation to take that oxygen to the brain, the brain is irreversibly damaged within 3 to 4 minutes. The purpose of BLS is to maintain an adequate ventilation and circulation until the underlying cause of the respiratory/cardiac arrest can be corrected. Usually, therefore, BLS will not revive a patient. However, it can help keep a patient alive until a defibrillator and advanced life support (ALS) procedures are available to correct the rhythm of the heart. Rarely, BLS may revive a patient if respiratory failure is the cause of collapse.

MANAGEMENT OF A COLLAPSED PATIENT

Follow the ABC of management for a patient who has collapsed.

A Assessment

If a patient has fainted, they will respond quickly to being laid flat. If they don't respond quickly, you must consider other causes of collapse. Assess the patient; make sure you - and they - are in a safe environment, away from any potential hazards. Shake them gently on the shoulder, call out their name and ask, "Are you all right?" If they do not respond, call for the help of other members of the practice staff. Depending on where you are will determine how you manage other patients in the practice. If you are in a public area, like the waiting room, try to get the other patients either to help you, by asking a particular individual to do a particular task (such as call for an ambulance) or get out of the way.

B Breathing

Next you should assess the airway. Maintaining a patent airway is very important in preventing any deterioration in the condition of an unconscious individual, including the onset of cardiac arrest.

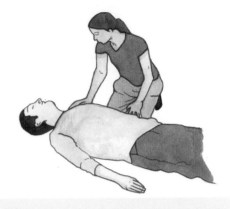

Figure 2.1. Shake and shout – "are you all right?"

Obstruction of the airway is common and is usually the result of the tongue falling back into the pharynx. In a dental setting other potential causes of airway obstruction are:

- vomit or blood
- foreign bodies - loose dentures or teeth
- oedema of the upper airway in anaphylaxis or angio-oedema
- bronchospasm (asthma)

Open the airway (Figure 2.2)

- Tilt the head back
- Lift the chin to open the airway
- Remove any visible obstruction from the victim's mouth, including dislodged dentures. Leave well fitting dentures in place.

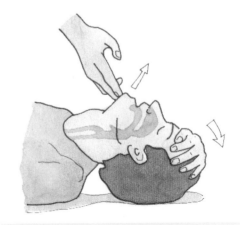

Figure 2.2. Open the airway - head tilt, chin lift

Assess the airway (*Figure 2.3*)

- **Look** - down the line of the chest to see if it rises and falls with inspiration and expiration
- **Listen** - at the mouth and nose for breathing sounds or the suggestion that there may be a blocked airway
- **Feel** - for expired air against your cheek

You are advised not to spend more than 10 seconds assessing if the patient is breathing

If the patient is <u>not breathing</u>

- Send for help. If alone, leave victim and go for help. Return and start rescue breathing (*Figure 2.5*).
- Give 2 slow, effective rescue breaths
    - Ensure head tilt and chin lift – to open the airway
    - Pinch the patient's nose
    - Take a deep breath, place your lips around the patient's mouth
    - Blow into the patient's mouth, watching to see that the chest rises
    - Take your mouth away from the patient and watch their chest fall
    - If there is difficulty achieving an effective rescue breath, make up to 5 attempts. Then move on even if unsuccessful.

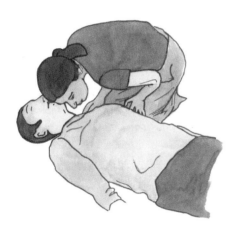

Figure 2.3. Look, listen and **feel** for signs of breathing

If the patient <u>is breathing</u>
- Turn into the recovery position (*Figure 2.4*)
- Send or go for help
- Check for continued breathing

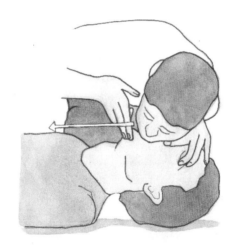

Figure 2.5. Rescue breathing (mouth to mouth ventilation)

C Circulation

Assess for signs of a circulation
- Check the carotid pulse
- Take no more than 10 seconds to do this

Feel for a carotid pulse in the neck. To palpate the carotid pulse, locate the thyroid cartilage (Adam's apple) with the tips of your fingers then move your fingers laterally into the depression either side of

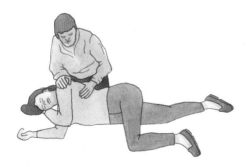

Figure 2.4. Recovery position

the thyroid cartilage and trachea. It is worth trying this on yourself or a colleague so you are in no doubt.

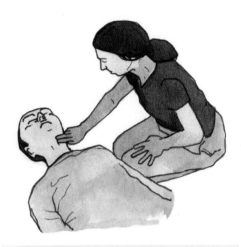

Figure 2.6. Feeling for a carotid pulse

If the patient has a circulation
- Continue rescue breathing (mouth to mouth) until the patient starts breathing on their own
- Check the circulation every 10 breaths
- If the patient starts to breathe normally but remains unconscious, turn them into the recovery position and continue to monitor breathing/circulation

If there are no signs of circulation
Start chest compressions
- 15 compressions followed by 2 rescue breaths
- Repeat until qualified help arrives or the patient shows signs of life

External cardiac massage (chest compressions) is very tiring but you should persist and only stop to recheck the circulation if the victim makes a movement or takes a breath.

Repeat the cardiac compressions aiming at a **rate of 100 per minute**. Whether you are a single 'rescuer' or if there are two or more of you, deliver two breaths of expired air per 15 cardiac compressions. This ratio is now

Chest Compressions
- Stand or kneel at the side of the patient, depending on whether they are on the dental chair or the floor
- Identify lower border of the ribs nearest you. Move your fingers along them toward the midline to locate the xiphisternum
- Place the heel of one hand two finger breadths above the lower border of the sternum (*Figure 2.7*)
- Place the heel of the other hand on top of the first and interlock the fingers of both hands
- Position yourself with your shoulders vertically above the patient's chest
- Keeping your arms straight, press down on the patient's sternum to depress it 4-5 cms

preferred as more cardiac compressions can be given each minute than under the previous guidance of one breath per five compressions. Furthermore, when chest compressions are performed during a cardiac arrest, the coronary perfusion pressure rises progressively with each compression and this perfusion pressure is lost each time cardiac massage is stopped to allow breaths to be given. Chest compressions rarely cause serious injury and the potential benefits of external cardiac massage outweigh any risks.

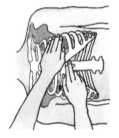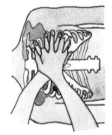

Figure 2.7. Position of the hands for chest compressions

USE OF AIRWAY ADJUNCTS
Expired air ventilation provides air containing 16% oxygen. The use of a ventilation mask, such as the Laerdal

'Pocket Mask', described in Section 1, avoids the need for mouth-to-mouth contact and the attendant concerns over cross-infection (*Figure 2.10*). It is best when using a ventilation mask to kneel above the patient's head. Place the mask over their nose and mouth and, with your fingers behind the ramus and angle of the mandible so effecting a jaw thrust, press the mask onto the skin of the face to form an air-tight seal. The one-way valve allows your expired air to pass to the patient while their expired air is directed away from you. There is an attachment on the mask which allows a supplementary oxygen supply to be added to enrich the expired air with which you are ventilating the patient.

If you are having difficulty maintaining the patency of the airway, consider the use of an oral (Guedal) airway (see Section 1). Other airway adjuncts, such as a bag and mask manual ventilator, can also assist ventilation and increase the oxygen concentration delivered to the lungs. These are discussed in more detail in Section 1.

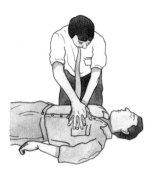

Figure 2.8. Single rescuer basic life support

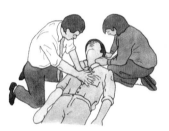

Figure 2.9. Two rescuer basic life support

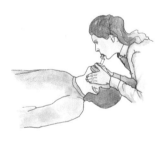

Figure 2.10. Pocket mask being used with a non-return valve

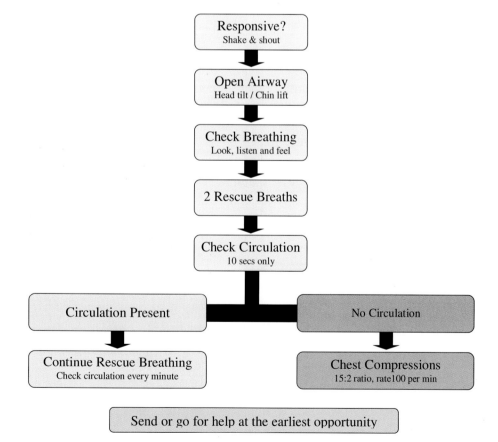

Responsive?
Shake & shout

Open Airway
Head tilt / Chin lift

Check Breathing
Look, listen and feel

2 Rescue Breaths

Check Circulation
10 secs only

| Circulation Present | No Circulation |

Continue Rescue Breathing
Check circulation every minute

Chest Compressions
15:2 ratio, rate 100 per min

Send or go for help at the earliest opportunity

Figure 2.11. Adult basic life support protocol

THE CHAIN OF SURVIVAL FOR CARDIAC ARREST

Although BLS will help to maintain a circulation, the heart is unlikely to resume a functional heartbeat without defibrillation. The prognosis for recovery from a cardiac arrest is best when defibrillation is carried out early. The chances of successful defibrillation are believed to be greatest within about 90 seconds of the onset of ventricular fibrillation, after which the chances of success fall by about 10% for every minute that defibrillation is delayed. This underlines the importance of calling for expert help sooner rather than later. The use of automatic external defibrillators (AED) (see Section 1 and *Figures 2.12, 2.13*) has simplified the process of defibrillation so that even lay people can perform defibrillation with minimal training. Where they are available, AEDs have significantly improved survival from cardiac arrest by reducing the time between arrest and defibrillation.

THE CHAIN OF SURVIVAL CONCEPT

The chance of surviving a cardiac arrest is considerably improved if the following steps are followed:

- Early recognition of cardiac arrest
- Early activation of emergency services
- Early basic life support
- Early defibrillation
- Early advanced life support

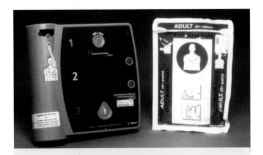

Figure 2.12. Automatic External Defibrillator (AED) with disposable electrode pads

---

AUTOMATIC EXTERNAL DEFIBRILLATORS (AED)

Protocol for AED use: (*Figure 2.14*)

If there is NO sign of a circulation:

- Perform BLS until AED is available
- Switch on AED and apply electrode pads to chest
- Follow spoken/visual directions
- Ensure nobody touches the patient while the AED analyses the rhythm

If a shock IS indicated

- Ensure everyone is clear of the patient
- Push the 'shock' button as directed
- Repeat 'analyse' or 'shock' as directed
- Do not perform pulse checks between the first 3 shocks
- After 3 shocks check circulation

  If NO circulation

  - Perform CPR for 1 minute (most AEDs will automatically time this)
  - Stop CPR and 'analyse' rhythm (most AEDs will automatically initiate this)
  - Continue the AED algorithm as directed by the AED voice and visual prompts

  If signs of circulation ARE present

  - Check for breathing
  - If breathing present, put in recovery position
  - If no breathing, start rescue breathing and re-check circulation every minute

  If NO shock is indicated

  - Check for signs of circulation
  - If no circulation – continue as above

  You should continue to follow AED instructions until advanced life support (ALS) is available

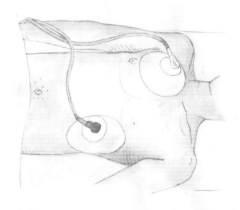

Figure 2.13. AED pads on patient

ADVANCED LIFE SUPPORT

Defibrillation may be even more effective if performed by someone with advanced life support (ALS) training. ALS training includes training in the different causes of cardiac arrest and the administration of emergency drugs in a cardiac arrest. ALS training and the use of ALS drugs are outside the remit of this book. However, those dentists who are interested are encouraged to obtain ALS training as it will increase their confidence and ability to deal with any emergency situation. Details of ALS training courses can be obtained from the Resuscitation Council (UK)[24].

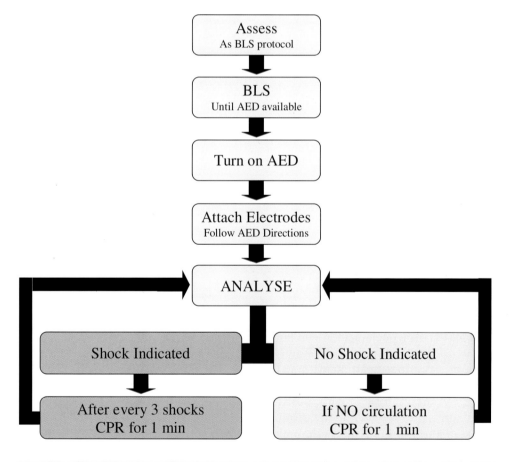

Figure 2.14. Automatic External Defibrillator (AED) protocol

MANAGEMENT OF COLLAPSE OF UNKNOWN CAUSE

By far the most common cause of loss of consciousness in a dental surgery is a simple faint (vaso-vagal syncope). This often occurs at the sight of a needle or after an injection and the precaution of lying the patient flat before administering local anaesthetic should prevent the patient from losing consciousness. Fainting is managed well in dental practice, judging by how few serious consequences have been reported.

MAIN CAUSES OF SUDDEN LOSS OF CONSCIOUSNESS IN THE DENTAL CHAIR

- Fainting
- Cardiac arrest
- Epilepsy
- Postural hypotension
- Hypoglycaemia
- Steroid insufficiency (Addisonian crisis)
- Anaphylaxis
- Stroke

Other less common causes of collapse may be suggested by the medical history. If a patient who is a known insulin-dependent diabetic collapses, it may well be the result of hypoglycaemia; similarly, collapse of a patient with a history of angina or a previous heart attack may be caused by a myocardial infarct. A known epileptic may lose consciousness immediately prior to a fit. The clinical features of an episode of collapse may also aid diagnosis; for example, severe chest pain preceding collapse suggests myocardial infarction, while facial swelling and an urticarial rash suggest an allergic reaction.

A patient will usually become unwell before losing consciousness and you should look out for any signs that may suggest a cause. The patient's medical history can be crucial

in this regard, hence the importance of updating it at every recall.

However, the cause of a collapse is not always immediately obvious and in such circumstances it is important to work quickly to exclude cardiac arrest and identify the cause so that it can be managed appropriately before the patient's condition deteriorates. This is not easy in an emergency and it is important to think through in advance how such a situation should be dealt with. In the box (p23) we suggest a protocol for managing such a patient.

Unconsciousness is the result of cerebral hypoxia. If this is prolonged it will lead to respiratory and cardiac arrest. It is essential, therefore to monitor the pulse and respiration of an unconscious person and start artificial ventilation or chest compressions immediately should either respiratory or cardiac arrest occur.

SUGGESTED PROTOCOL FOR MANAGEMENT OF COLLAPSE OF UNKNOWN CAUSE

First principle: Exclude the commonest cause (faint) and most serious (cardiac arrest) then attempt to manage accordingly.

- Lay the patient flat with the feet slightly raised (Trendelenburg position); if the cause of collapse is a faint, recovery will be rapid.
- Ask the patient if they are all right – 'shake and shout'

If recovery is NOT rapid
- Consider other causes of collapse, which may be suspected from the medical history or signs and symptoms, especially
    - cardiac arrest
    - (diabetic) hypoglycaemia
    - anaphylaxis
- Call for help from other members of the practice staff
- Open airway. Check breathing – look, listen, feel

If they are NOT breathing
- Give TWO 'rescue' breaths of mouth to mouth ventilation
- Check for a pulse. Take no more than 10 seconds to do this
- Get someone to call an ambulance by dialling 999

If NO pulse
- Start chest compressions
- Continue **basic life support** until help arrives
- Defibrillate at the earliest opportunity

If the patient is unconscious but IS breathing and HAS a pulse

There are several possible causes. Hypoglycaemia is one of the more likely and treating the collapse as if it were a hypoglycaemic episode has few risks, so give either:
- Glucagon 1unit (1mg) i/m

or
- Glucose 50ml of 20% sterile solution by slow i/v injection, if you can gain venous access.

Put the patient in the recovery position, monitor their airway and give oxygen. A hypoglycaemic patient should improve within a few minutes with this regimen.

An unconscious patient should be monitored closely at all times to ensure that cardiac arrest does not supervene

If there is still no improvement

Consider an Addisonian crisis; again treatment has few risks:
- Give 200mg hydrocortisone i/m or i/v
- Continue to monitor airway and circulation throughout and give oxygen

Other causes of collapse, e.g. epilepsy, are usually evident from the physical signs. You should seek urgent medical assistance for any cause of collapse that does not respond quickly to treatment.

3

MANAGEMENT OF THE CAUSES OF COLLAPSE

INTRODUCTION

In Section 2 we covered basic life support, the chain of survival for cardiac arrest and the management of the patient who collapses where there is no indication of the cause. In this section we cover the different medical emergencies that commonly lead to collapse of the patient and loss of consciousness. In most cases, information from the medical history or the patient's signs and symptoms, will provide some indication of the cause of the collapse. In such cases, rapid treatment will usually revive the patient or prevent the patient's condition deteriorating into cardiac arrest.

For each condition we provide a scenario to give an example of how such an emergency might arise in the dental surgery. We also discuss the causes, signs and symptoms, prevention and management of the condition as well as providing additional background information where appropriate.

FAINTING

CLINICAL SCENARIO

David Kronkowski is a 23-year-old rugby playing welder. He is an irregular dental attender but has had a toothache for the last three days. He has been ruminating about today's appointment, slept badly last night and missed breakfast. It's a warm day.

On entering the surgery he appears a little anxious but denies feeling in any way nervous on questioning. He sits in the dental chair and upon being asked to open his mouth wide, he catches sight of the local anaesthetic syringe, grips the handles of the chair, breaks out into a sweat, becomes pale and a glazed look comes over his eyes. He faints. What would you do next?

CAUSES

Predisposing factors include anxiety, pain, fatigue, fasting and a high environmental temperature or humidity. It is particularly common in young men.

SIGNS AND SYMPTOMS

Signs and symptoms of an impending faint include:

- Dizziness
- Yawning
- Nausea
- Pallor
- Cold moist skin
- Slow, weak pulse

The patient then loses consciousness: they may convulse, particularly if there is any delay in treating the cerebral hypoxia

---

PREVENTION

A history of previous fainting should not be ignored. Predisposing factors should be minimised and patients should be encouraged to eat normally prior to their

---

MANAGEMENT

- In the dental chair, position the patient in a flat, slightly head down position (Trendelenburg position), otherwise lay them flat on the ground
- Loosen any tight clothing around the neck
- Monitor pulse and respiration

---

appointment and wear comfortable, cool clothing whilst in the dental chair. Furthermore, prevention is always better than cure: if patients are given injections when they are lying down, they will not faint!

Recovery is normally quick and accompanied by a rapid and full pulse. The patient should be reassured and given some form of glucose or a sugary drink to raise the blood glucose before continuing with treatment.

If the patient does not recover rapidly after being laid flat:

- Consider other causes of collapse
- Call for help
- Check airway and circulation – **start basic life support**

BACKGROUND INFORMATION[25,26]

Fainting is by far the most common cause of sudden loss of consciousness in the dental surgery. The exact mechanism of, or reason for, the fainting reflex is not clear. In response to apprehension or anxiety about a situation, there is preparation for 'fight or flight' with an increase in pulse rate and blood pressure along with cold sweating and pallor, all of which are associated with activation of the sympathetic nervous system and adrenal medulla. Paradoxically, there is then a sudden and profound reversal of these effects, with slowing of the heart rate and a fall in blood pressure; it is these inappropriate 'vasovagal' effects, which seem completely illogical and have yet to be fully explained, that result in loss of consciousness.

There also appears to be an association with a low blood sugar that reverses spontaneously within a short time after the faint. This hypoglycaemia, combined with the fall in blood pressure, may well be responsible for the sudden loss of consciousness. From experience we all know that many patients who faint have missed a meal prior to attending the dental surgery; they seem to improve after they have been given glucose or a sugary drink to the extent that, more often than not, the proposed treatment can be carried out.

CARDIAC ARREST

CLINICAL SCENARIO

Mr Tuoparis is 57 years old and attending your surgery for adjustment of a recently fitted upper denture. He is late. The traffic was bad. He had difficulty finding a parking space, which was quite a long way from the surgery, and had to jog to make up time. He is perspiring and breathless when he arrives and sits in the waiting room gasping for breath. He does not look very well. His breathing does not get any easier while he is waiting and he fumbles around in his pockets for his glyceryl trinitrate spray. Eventually he finds it and sprays it into his mouth. It does not appear to make any difference; he is sweating, gasping for breath, his skin is ashen coloured and he appears to be in pain. Your receptionist is worried and calls you out of the surgery. You are immediately concerned and help him into an empty surgery. He tells you that he is having a lot of pain in his chest, a crushing pain. You ask your nurse to get the oxygen and she looks blankly at you. You rush out to the receptionist and ask her to get the oxygen. She brings it to the surgery and you put the mask over the patient's nose and mouth and turn it on full. He is complaining of terrible pain in his chest and is panicking; he collapses. What would you do next?
This patient is having a myocardial infarct, which has lead to a cardiac arrest......

CAUSES

Sudden cessation of an effective heart beat results in acute failure of cardiac output (circulatory failure). There are four causes:

- Ventricular fibrillation (VF)

- Pulseless ventricular tachycardia (VT)

- Pulseless electrical activity (PEA)

- Asystole

In ventricular fibrillation (VF) and pulseless ventricular tachycardia (VT), the heart beats rapidly and ineffectually; these are the commonest causes of cardiac arrest and carry the best prognosis as they are amenable to defibrillation. On an electrocardiogram (ECG), these appear as irregular waveforms (*Figure 3.1*) which reduce in amplitude as they progress into asystole which is not amenable to defibrillation. In pulseless electrical activity (PEA) there is a severe reduction in

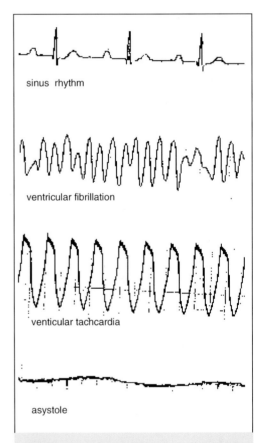

sinus rhythm

ventricular fibrillation

venticular tachcardia

asystole

Figure 3.1. ECG rhythms

the heart's output, which is clinically indistinguishable from cardiac arrest but with normal, or near normal, electrical activity as would be seen on an ECG. It is very unlikely that cardiac arrest due to PEA would occur in a dental setting.

SIGNS AND SYMPTOMS
Cardiac arrest may complicate myocardial infarction, thus:

- Signs and symptoms of myocardial infarction preceding loss of consciousness
    - Chest pain
    - Shortness of breath
    - Sweating
    - Nausea
- Sudden loss of consciousness
- Pallor and irregular or absent respiration in a collapsed patient
- <u>Absent pulse</u> - palpate the carotid artery in the neck anterior to the sternomastoid

Late signs
- Cyanosis
- Dilatation of the pupils and absent light reflex
- Unmeasurable blood pressure

In the dental surgery, ventricular fibrillation or asystole most commonly result from:

- Myocardial infarction
- Hypoxia
- Severe hypotension

- Anaesthetic overdose
- Drug overdose
- Respiratory arrest
- Pulmonary embolism
- Other causes of collapse

PREVENTION
Avoid stress, particularly in patients with a history of previous myocardial infarction or cardiovascular disease. Take care to avoid respiratory depression or hypoxia. Manage promptly causes of collapse. These patients require specialist assessment before administering i/v sedation.

BACKGROUND INFORMATION[24, 27-29]
The automatic external defibrillator (AED) is a significant development in defibrillator technology. Conditions for defibrillation are often optimal for only a short period of time after the onset of the arrhythmia, so that any delay in defibrillation can be crucial. AEDs placed in large public buildings, emergency vehicles and aircraft have saved many lives by reducing the time between cardiac arrest and defibrillation.

In Las Vegas, security staff at casinos resuscitated 105 patients in ventricular fibrillation, of whom 56 (53%) survived to be discharged from hospital. Rapid identification of collapsed patients was achieved through the closed circuit television surveillance. Locating AEDs in other parts of the community where fewer arrests are witnessed are the subject of ongoing studies. In the U.K., the remoteness of rural communities can impede a quick response by the ambulance service. Increasingly, trained lay people (termed 'first responders') who live locally and are equipped with an AED, can be despatched by ambulance control at the same time as the ambulance, to provide defibrillation should it be required.

When using an AED several safety factors need to be borne in mind. Metal objects such as chains may cause minor skin burns if left in place on the front of the chest and should be removed. Any self-medication patches attached to the front of the patient's chest should also be removed. Oxygen should be directed away from the patient or turned off during defibrillation. Automatic external defibrillation is likely to develop as an important step in out of hospital resuscitation over the next few years and AEDs are likely to become more widely distributed as their price continues to fall.

MANAGEMENT
Follow the protocol for basic life support (Section 2):
- Check responsiveness – shake and shout
- In the dental chair - position head down. Otherwise, lay flat on the ground.
- Open airway - head tilt, chin lift
- Check breathing – look, listen, feel
- Give two 'rescue' breaths
- Assess circulation – if no circulation:
- Start chest compressions – follow **basic life support** protocol
- Defibrillate at earliest opportunity. If possible, initiate **advanced life support** procedures (see Section 2).

Call for help at the earliest opportunity and get someone to call for an ambulance. Give the emergency services as much information as you can and tell them that basic life support is being carried out.

POSTURAL HYPOTENSION

CLINICAL SCENARIO
Mrs Lopez is a 60-year-old lady who has a 90 minute appointment for two fillings and a bridge prep. She is generally well but takes medication for high blood pressure. Everything has gone well and you have just cemented the temporary bridge. While you write the notes, your nurse puts the chair back up and helps Mrs Lopez from the chair. She turns to talk to you and then stumbles and collapses on the floor. What would you do next?

CAUSES
Some patients are unable to compensate quickly for the fall in blood pressure that occurs on standing. As a result, when they rise quickly from a lying position, blood pools in their legs and the brain suffers a temporary lack of oxygen that may result in loss of consciousness. This is most likely to occur:

- After prolonged periods lying down

- In the elderly

- In those taking anti-hypertensive drugs

- In diabetics.

SIGNS AND SYMPTOMS
• Pallor
• Unsteadiness
• Collapse
Prompted by standing up quickly from a supine or seated position

PREVENTION
It can be prevented in susceptible patients by moving them gradually from lying to standing. Manage postural hypotension as if it were a faint.

MANAGEMENT
• In the dental chair - position head down. Otherwise, lay flat on the ground
• Recovery should be rapid
• When fully recovered, slowly move the patient from supine to sitting
• Let the patient rest for a while in a sitting position
• Slow transition to standing

BACKGROUND INFORMATION
The control of blood pressure on moving from supine to standing is mainly under the control of the baroreceptor reflex. On standing, the blood pressure in the carotid sinus falls due to pooling of blood in the lower extremities. Baroreceptor nerve activity is reduced and the brain stem responds by increased sympathetic activity which results in vasoconstriction and an increased heart rate. Together these correct the fall in blood pressure at the carotid sinus.

This response may be sluggish in the elderly and those on drugs that modulate vascular tone or heart rate. Autonomic neuropathy in diabetics may also reduce the effectiveness of the baroreceptor response.

HYPOGLYCAEMIA

CLINICAL SCENARIO

Diane Philips, a 30-year-old insulin dependent diabetic, is attending your practice this morning for some routine restorative work. She got up late and, while she gave herself her normal dose of insulin, in the rush to get her children to school, she ate only half a slice of toast. At the practice, your current patient's extraction has turned into a difficult surgical and you are running late. In the waiting room, Mrs. Jones becomes anxious and confused. She is sweating and her hands are trembling. She asks for a sugary drink but collapses in the waiting room before this can be provided. This patient is having a hypoglycaemic episode. What would you do next?

CAUSES

Hypoglycaemia most often occurs in a known 'Type I' (insulin dependent) diabetic who has taken a normal dose of insulin but failed to eat adequately or at the right time. As a result the blood glucose levels fall to a low level (hypoglycaemia) and the brain is starved of glucose. First line emergency treatment of diabetics is therefore aimed at increasing blood glucose levels.

SIGNS AND SYMPTOMS

In a known diabetic, the following suggest hypoglycaemia - especially if a meal is known to have been missed:

- Increasing drowsiness
- Disorientation and confusion
- Excitability or aggressiveness
- Slurred speech

The sympathetic nervous system may be activated in an attempt to release more glucose. Consequently, autonomic symptoms include:

- Shaking
- Sweating
- Palpitations
- Anxiety and pallor

Hypoglycaemia can be quickly confirmed by measuring the blood glucose using a test reagent strip (e.g. Dextrostix®), if these are available. A diabetic may carry their own test system with them. Normal blood glucose is in the range 3.9 – 6.2mmol/L. Cognitive dysfunction develops at a glucose concentration around 3mmol/L and autonomic symptoms at around 2mmol/L.

PREVENTION

Give patients appointments early in a session, ensure that they are treated on time and not kept waiting. Avoid treating at mealtimes. Enquire whether they have had their normal food and insulin intake. If not, give a sugary drink prior to commencing any treatment (even now, many patients mistakenly believe that they need to starve prior to a local anaesthetic).

MANAGEMENT

If conscious, give glucose or sugar orally as either:

- 50g Glucose dissolved in water to make a drink
- Hypostop® - a gel preparation which contains glucose
- Lucozade® or another soft drink (not the 'diet' variety)
- Dextrosol® tablets or at least four sugar lumps

If unconscious, give either:

- Glucagon 1mg by i/m, s/c or i/v injection
- 50ml of 20% sterile glucose by slow i/v injection

Lay the patient in the recovery position

If recovery is not rapid:

- Consider other causes of collapse
- Call for help
- Check airway and circulation – if necessary start **basic life support**

It should be remembered that diabetics may also faint or suffer from other types of medical emergency. They have an increased risk of a myocardial infarction or stroke as atherosclerosis is a common complication of longstanding diabetes.

Notes: Sugar (sucrose, a combination of glucose and fructose) takes longer to act than glucose. Glucagon, given by intramuscular injection, is simple and safe to use. Rarely, however, it can be ineffective in protracted hypoglycaemia or if hepatic glycogen stores are depleted. 50ml of 20% glucose solution given intravenously produces a rapid response. Alternatively, 25ml of 50% glucose solution may be given. However, the stronger the solution used the more viscous it is and the more difficult it is to inject. Viscous glucose solutions are best administered through a large bore (white) needle into a large vein in the anti-cubital fossa. If hypoglycaemia has been caused by an oral antidiabetic drug (rare), the patient should be admitted to hospital.

BACKGROUND INFORMATION[30-32]

Diabetes mellitus is a common disease, characterised by raised blood glucose levels, and affects over 30 million people worldwide. Normally, blood glucose levels are regulated by the release of insulin from the pancreatic islet cells, which lowers blood glucose. Diabetes mellitus results either from failure of insulin production (Type I, insulin dependent diabetes) or from a relative insensitivity of the tissues to the effects of insulin (Type II, insulin independent diabetes). Type II diabetes is becoming more common with the increase in obesity in Western populations and is now being reported in juveniles for the first time.

There is considerable variation in the severity of the signs and symptoms of hypoglycaemia between diabetics and sometimes the symptoms will not be recognised by the patient, requiring relatives and dental practitioners to be alert to the warning signs.

Several important studies published in the last decade have confirmed that careful glycaemic control in diabetics results in delay and possibly even prevention of the long-term complications of diabetes. With this knowledge, it is likely that poorly controlled non-insulin dependent diabetics will increasingly be treated with insulin, while insulin dependent diabetics will be encouraged to adopt tighter glycaemic control. As control becomes tighter, the potential for hypoglycaemic episodes increases and thus diabetics and their dental practitioners are increasingly likely to encounter such episodes.

HYPERGLYCAEMIA

In an undiagnosed diabetic, or a diabetic who fails to take their treatment, blood glucose levels may rise to high levels (hyperglycaemia). Although this can result in coma, it is of much slower onset than hypoglycaemic coma and is unlikely to present in the dental surgery. In any case, it is better to assume that a diabetic in difficulty is suffering a hypoglycaemic episode and treat it as such. Giving glucose to a hypoglycaemic diabetic will save their life and will not seriously worsen the prognosis of a hyperglycaemic one.

STEROID INSUFFICIENCY (ADDISONIAN CRISIS)

CLINICAL SCENARIO

Alison Jones is a 30-year-old printer. On her medical history form she lists Addison's disease, for which she takes hydrocortisone and fludrocortisone. She is attending your surgery today for surgical removal of a wisdom tooth under local anaesthetic. Her previous appointment, when the tooth removal was discussed, had been rushed as you were running late. As a result, she was not sure if you were going to use local or general anaesthetic and she has starved herself this morning and not taken her regular medication. On her arrival today you forgot to check her medical history and ten minutes into bone removal, she becomes unconscious. What would you do next?

CAUSES

The natural production of adrenocortical steroids is increased at times of physiological stress and is important in maintaining blood pressure and blood glucose levels. In Addison's disease (primary hypoadrenocorticism) there is adrenal atrophy, often the result of auto-antibodies to the adrenal cortex, and failure of adrenocortical production of cortisol and aldosterone. More commonly, steroid insufficiency is the result of long-term systemic steroid therapy. Systemic steroids inhibit adrenocorticotrophic hormone (ACTH) production by the pituitary gland. Without ACTH stimulation, the adrenal cortex atrophies and may eventually become incapable of producing an increase in cortisol production at times of stress. With prolonged use of topical or inhaled steroids, there may be sufficient systemic absorption to cause adrenal insufficiency. It is worth enquiring of the patient's doctor or hospital specialist if this is likely. In general the longer the course of steroid treatment and the higher the dose used, the more likely the adrenal response to stress will be suppressed.

SIGNS AND SYMPTOMS
- Pallor
- Rapid, weak or impalpable pulse
- Loss of consciousness
- Rapidly falling blood pressure
- Failure to regain consciousness when laid flat

PREVENTION

Always check the medical history and give steroid cover to any patients undergoing surgery or another stressful procedure who have been on a long-term course of steroids during the previous 12 months. Steroid cover should also be considered for patients who have been on long term high dose steroid therapy within the last two years and need to undergo anything more than minor surgery. Patients taking systemic steroids should carry a steroid card with them detailing their treatment.

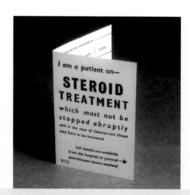

Figure 3.2. Steroid card

Steroid Cover

For minor surgery (e.g. biopsy or single extraction):

- Double normal oral steroid dose on the morning of the procedure

Or give

- 50mg hydrocortisone i/m 30 mins before, or i/v immediately before the procedure

For major surgery or trauma (e.g. maxillofacial surgery):

- 100mg hydrocortisone i/m 30 mins before, or i/v immediately before the procedure and then 6 hourly for up to 72 hours

---

MANAGEMENT

Even if the cause of collapse is unclear, it is safest to give corticosteroids immediately

- Lay the patient flat and raise their legs
- Open the airway
- Give 200mg hydrocortisone sodium succinate i/v (or i/m). Repeat if necessary.
- Give oxygen
- Call an ambulance
- Monitor patient

Consider other possible causes of collapse

BACKGROUND INFORMATION[33-36]
Among the body's responses to surgery are an increase in plasma concentrations of adrenocorticotrophic hormone (ACTH) and cortisol. After minor surgery the increase is minimal in most people. However, the ability to respond is totally lost in those who have had an adrenalectomy and in some patients with Addison's disease. In patients taking oral corticosteroids, the ability to respond to surgery is suppressed. The corticosteroid dose below which adrenal suppression is unlikely to occur is difficult to predict but suppression has not been reported with doses below 5mg of prednisolone a day.

Various perioperative corticosteroid replacement regimes have been proposed for use in general surgery and these have frequently been adopted for use in oral surgery. The traditional regime followed the initial reports of fatal peri-operative adrenal suppression in the 1950s and involved high dose corticosteroid cover. Whilst such regimes have had few adverse effects, concerns have been raised that such high dose regimes are unnecessary and may impair wound healing, cause an increased susceptibility to infection and cause disruption of control in insulin-dependent diabetics.

In recent years, several small studies investigating adrenal function in patients undergoing surgery have been undertaken. These involved patients on daily oral doses of 10mg prednisolone or less, and found no evidence of adrenocorticosteroid insufficiency. As a result, a more recent alternative approach to corticosteroid replacement for general surgery takes into account the dose and duration of maintenance corticosteroid therapy, and the nature of the surgery. These regimes involve far lower doses of steroid cover than previously given. There are no definitive guidelines for oral surgery in patients taking oral corticosteroids, but the physiological stress involved is likely to be no more severe than minor general surgical operations. In the few documented cases of apparent adrenal crisis during dental surgery, several additional factors have been identified which could have increased the risk of developing hypotension. These include the use of general anaesthetic, multiple extractions, oral infection and hypovolaemia. It is therefore unlikely that a routine extraction under local anaesthetic in a patient taking low dose systemic corticosteroids will precipitate an adrenal crisis. The difficulty in performing prospective randomised studies however, means that a consensus on this issue is still being developed.

ANAPHYLAXIS

CLINICAL SCENARIO

Kevin McGrath is a 42-year-old builder. He doesn't like dentists or doctors and, even though he suffered with rheumatic fever and subsequent heart valve damage as a teenager, he tends to steer clear of all matters to do with health as much as he can. He had a reaction to penicillin, a rash on his hands and arms, a number of years ago but thought nothing of it. It went away when he stopped taking the tablets.

He's been having discomfort from a periodontally involved molar for a couple of months and has decided to get it sorted out. He attended your practice last week. From your questioning about his medical history, you managed to glean that he has had rheumatic fever with heart valve damage and decide that he will need antibiotic cover to remove the uncomfortable molar. You were interrupted by a phone call from home as you were asking about allergies, to which he gave you a rather vague answer, and you forgot to come back to the subject when you returned.

He returns today for the treatment under antibiotic cover. Your nurse gives him 3 grammes of amoxicillin without any further questions about allergies. After about five minutes, while sitting in the waiting room, he begins to feel uncomfortable with general itching and a bit of a rash developing on his hands. He ignores it at first but then starts to have difficulty breathing. The receptionist is concerned about his appearance and calls you to see him. His face is starting to swell and he looks flushed, he is having obvious difficulty breathing and is wheezing. You feel his pulse, which is rapid and weak. He loses consciousness. This person is having a severe allergic (anaphylactic) reaction. What would you do next?

CAUSES

There is a spectrum of allergic reactions and anaphylaxis is the most severe. It is caused by the massive release of histamine from mast cells when they are exposed to a foreign antigen to which they have become sensitised (Type I hypersensitivity). The release of histamine increases vascular permeability and causes vasodilatation which leads to oedema, flushing and a sudden fall in blood pressure. It also causes broncho-constriction resulting in wheezing and difficulty in breathing. In anaphylaxis, the degree of respiratory difficulty and hypotension produced are life threatening.

Drugs are the most common cause of anaphylaxis in the dental surgery, particularly penicillin (including amoxicillin). However, a growing number of individuals are allergic to other materials used in the dental practice, notably latex (natural rubber).

In general the more rapid the onset of an allergic reaction, the more profound it tends to be.

SIGNS AND SYMPTOMS

Anaphylactic shock usually occurs within a few minutes of exposure to the allergen, but it may be delayed for 30 minutes or more. Features include:

- Facial flushing, swelling or itching
- Paraesthesia
- Generalised urticaria or itching
- Wheezing and difficulty breathing
- Loss of consciousness
- A rapid, weak or impalpable pulse
- Falling blood pressure
- Pallor progressing to cyanosis
- Finally, cardiac arrest

PREVENTION

Take a careful medical history of any allergies. These patients often have a history of allergy or atopy (eczema, hay fever or asthma). Avoid exposing them to any known allergens.

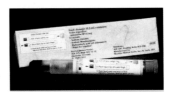

Figure 3.3. Patient operated epinephrine (adrenaline) auto-injector

MANAGEMENT

If respiratory distress is the major feature:

- Keep patient in the most comfortable position for breathing (usually sitting up)

However, if they lose consciousness or become hypotensive:

- Lay them flat with legs raised

In all cases:

- Maintain the airway and give oxygen
- Give 0.5mL of 1:1,000 (500µg) epinephrine (adrenaline) i/m* [For children 6 months - 6 years 0.12mL, 6-12 years 0.25mL and >12 years old 0.5mL]
- Repeat after 5 minutes if no improvement
- Call an ambulance

Supplementary medication:

- Chlorphenamine (formerly chlorpheniramine) (Piriton®) 10-20mg by i/m or slow i/v injection
- Hydrocortisone, 200mg i/v or i/m
- If available, i/v fluids will help restore the blood pressure

* 1 ml of 1: 1,000 epinephrine (adrenaline) Min-I-Jet® pre-loaded syringes are available with a 21 gauge 1.5" needle for i/m injection. I/m epinephrine is quickly absorbed, safe and predictable. Patients with a history of anaphylaxis may carry their own auto-injector epinephrine devices (*Figure 3.3*) e.g. EpiPen® or Anapen®. These dispense 300µg of epinephrine.

BACKGROUND INFORMATION[37-41]

The incidence of acute anaphylaxis appears to be increasing in the UK. Therapeutic drugs, especially antibiotics, remain an important cause, resulting in over half of the hospital admissions of patients with anaphylaxis.

Perhaps surprisingly, anaphylaxis is often poorly recognised by clinicians. The reasons include the varied clinical manifestations of anaphylaxis and the rarity of presentation. In 2002 the UK Resuscitation Council produced new guidelines for the emergency treatment of anaphylaxis. The guidelines are based predominantly on clinical experience, as there is a paucity of evidence on which to draw. The guidelines emphasise the importance of administering epinephrine (adrenaline) by the intramuscular route. They specifically advise against trying to give epinephrine subcutaneously as absorption is too slow and unreliable.

Epinephrine is an α and β receptor agonist. As an α receptor agonist, it reverses peripheral vasodilatation and reduces oedema. As a β receptor agonist, it dilates the airways, increases the force of myocardial contraction and suppresses the release of histamine and leukotrienes. Patients taking β blockers may not respond as effectively to epinephrine. In these cases supplementary medication may be of most value.

The anti-histamine chlorphenamine (chlorpheniramine) and hydrocortisone are useful adjuncts to epinephrine in the treatment of anaphylaxis. Hydrocortisone may be more valuable than once thought in supporting the action of epinephrine and continuing to act when the effect of epinephrine has worn off. It is particularly beneficial in severe or recurrent reactions and in patients with asthma. Hypovolaemia and hypotension are important features of anaphylaxis and infusion of intravenous fluids can be important in correcting these.

Occasionally a panic attack or a faint may be mistaken for an anaphylactic reaction. Victims of previous anaphylaxis may be particularly prone to panic attacks if they think they have been re-exposed to the allergen that caused the problem. If the reaction is hysterical rather than actual, there will be no hypotension, wheeze, urticarial rash or swelling.

See also the later sections on "angio-oedema" and "adverse reactions to local anaesthetic or other injections".

EPILEPSY

CLINICAL SCENARIO

Joe Amaechi, a 28-year-old epileptic, has recently stopped taking the medication prescribed to control his epilepsy; it makes him feel sleepy and very drowsy after he has had a couple of beers. He has had toothache for the last three days and has been kept awake with the pain. He is due to see you this afternoon for an extraction. While in the dental chair, after you have given an inferior dental block, he acts oddly. He tells you that he is not feeling well; he is very pale and almost immediately loses consciousness. He becomes completely rigid in a grotesque extended posture and lets out a cry. He starts to become cyanosed and after a few seconds starts jerking. He is having a grand mal epileptic attack. What would you do next?

CAUSES

In a known epileptic, fits may be precipitated by flashing lights, starvation, menstruation, stress or drugs such as methohexitone, tricyclic anti-depressants or alcohol. They may also occur due to cerebral hypoxia if there is delay in treating a patient who has fainted.

SIGNS AND SYMPTOMS OF A *GRAND MAL* ATTACK (*Figure 3.4*)

- An aura may precede the attack
- Sudden loss of consciousness
- Rigid extended appearance of the body as the extensor muscles of the body contract – this is the tonic phase
- The patient may give a cry as air is expelled past the tensed vocal cords and become cyanotic due to the cessation of breathing

After about 30 seconds

- Convulsions - generalised jerking movements – the clonic phase
- The patient may bite their tongue, froth at the mouth and be incontinent of urine
- Convulsions usually last a few minutes
- The patient may then become flaccid but remain unconscious for some time
- On regaining consciousness, the patient may be confused for some time (post-ictal confusion)

STATUS EPILEPTICUS

Status epilepticus, extended bouts of fitting or repeated episodes without the patient regaining consciousness, is an emergency that requires urgent control. Mortality may be as high as 10% as the epileptic activity may outstrip metabolic capacity and there may be severe cerebral hypoxia.

PREVENTION

Ensure a known epileptic has taken their prescribed medication. Minimise stress and avoid flashing lights, starvation and other risk factors, such as alcohol and some drugs (methohexitone and tricyclic antidepressants are epileptogenic). In a poorly controlled epileptic it may be worth placing an i/v cannula before carrying out a particularly stressful procedure or electing to perform the treatment under i/v sedation (with midazolam).

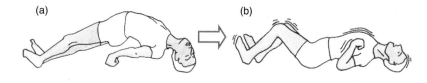

Figure 3.4. Epilepsy (a) tonic phase (b) clonic phase

MANAGEMENT

- Prevent the patient from injuring themselves - clear a space around them and lay them flat
- Do not attempt to put anything in the mouth or between the teeth to protect the tongue
- Put them in the recovery position
- Allow the patient to recover

If the convulsions do not stop or are repeated rapidly - this is **status epilepticus:**

- Maintain the airway
- Call an ambulance – the patient will require stabilisation in hospital
- Give up to 10mg diazepam (Diazemuls®) i/v or per rectum (see below)
- Give oxygen and monitor respiration
- Repeat diazepam if there is no recovery within 5 minutes

BACKGROUND INFORMATION[42-45]

Epilepsy is the result of abnormal paroxysmal discharge of cerebral nerve cells. Grand mal epilepsy (generalised convulsions) is the commonest type of epilepsy and is the type described above. There are other types which are unlikely to cause problems in the dental surgery; these include petit mal epilepsy, which is seen in children and is characterised by 'absences' which may mimic a faint, and temporal lobe epilepsy. Epilepsy may affect up to 2% of the general population and is more prevalent in the young and those with a mental or physical handicap. In most cases the epilepsy has no identifiable cause but it may be secondary to a number of other conditions affecting the brain and is a prominent feature of drug withdrawal. It can be difficult to diagnose and it is estimated that up to a quarter of patients are mislabelled as epileptics when they are not. Diagnosis is important as epileptics are often prevented from driving and may be committed to a lifetime of taking anticonvulsant drugs, such as carbamazepine, phenytoin and sodium valproate. These drugs have unpleasant side effects such as dizziness, drowsiness, gingival hypertrophy, acne, excessive growth of facial hair, which may deter patients from taking them.

Status epilepticus is a potentially fatal form of epilepsy in which the tonic and clonic phases alternate repeatedly without the patient regaining consciousness. It requires prompt treatment with a benzodiazepine, such as diazepam, administered intravenously or per rectum. The treatment of status epilepticus in a dental surgery setting has been a source of discussion. While the use of intravenous diazepam is theoretically sensible, concerns have been raised about the practicality of dentists trying to obtain venous access in an emergency on a fitting patient. Diazepam given per rectum is an alternative route used in hospital practice, although again in a dental practice situation some dentists may feel uncomfortable about using this route. There may also be problems with access, especially in heavier individuals. Recent interest has centred on the use of midazolam administered in the mouth where the route of absorption is via the buccal mucosa. Concerns have been raised about the risk of aspiration but because of the small volume and rapid absorption of midazolam by this route, it has been successfully used without problems in some epileptic patients. Further work is required but this does offer the possibility of an attractive alternative route of administration for benzodiazepines in patients in status epilepticus.

STROKE (CEREBRO-VASCULAR ACCIDENT)

CLINICAL SCENARIO

Geoffrey Greenwood, a 73-year-old retired draughtsman, attends your surgery today to have a couple of teeth out and an immediate denture fitted. From his medical history you know that he has longstanding hypertension, has maturity onset (type II) diabetes and has had an occasional transient ischaemic attack (TIA). On arriving at reception he says that he feels a bit off colour. The receptionist takes him to the staff room. When you see him, he has developed weakness of his right arm and leg and his speech is slurred. He is suffering a stroke. What do you do next?

CAUSES

Stroke is the result of sudden death, or hypoxia, of an area of brain tissue following haemorrhage or ischaemia. It can result from an intra-cranial haemorrhage, which distorts and tears apart the tissue or from thrombosis or an embolus which cuts off the blood supply to a part of the brain. The clinical picture is no guide to the underlying pathology.

SIGNS AND SYMPTOMS

- There may initially be a headache
- Sudden onset of difficulty in speech or swallowing
- Sudden onset of weakness of the limbs on one side of the body
- Sudden onset of paralysis of one side of the body (hemiplegia)
- Sudden loss of consciousness

PREVENTION

As it is likely to be a random event, there is little that can be done to prevent a stroke from occurring in the dental setting.

BACKGROUND INFORMATION[46-47]

Cerebrovascular accident (stroke) is the commonest neurological disease in the western world and the third most

---

MANAGEMENT

There is little that can be done in the dental surgery but:

- Maintain the airway
- Give oxygen
- Monitor the patient
- Call for an ambulance

---

common cause of death after heart disease and cancer. Strokes usually occur in patients over the age of 40 and are slightly more common in males. They are usually of rapid onset, develop over a matter of minutes and result in various neurological deficits (usually weakness of the limbs on one side) up to and including loss of consciousness, according to the part and extent of the brain affected. The death rate following a stroke is around 25% while around 40% will make a full recovery. The term 'transient ischaemic attack' (TIA) describes a localised neurological deficit lasting no more than 24 hours. Such events indicate an increased risk of future strokes or myocardial infarcts. Strokes occur as a result of haemorrhage from a cerebral blood vessel or occlusion of a vessel, leading to ischaemia of the surrounding brain, due to a thrombus or embolus.

Until recently, there was little to offer victims in the way of effective drug treatment to reverse the effects of a stroke. Recently, however, there has been interest in the use of intravenous tissue plasminogen activators to dissolve thromboses causing ischaemic strokes. For these drugs to be effective, patients need to be assessed rapidly and the drugs administered within three hours of the stroke. The use of thrombolysis is growing in the United States and may become more common in the UK over the next few years. Aspirin can help reduce the risk of early recurrent ischaemic stroke when given within 48 hours of a stroke. Unlike its use in myocardial infarction, however, there is little evidence that it should be administered prior to the patient reaching hospital.

4

INTRODUCTION

In this section we deal with those medical emergencies where the patient is usually conscious and where consciousness can usually be maintained with careful management. Again, for each condition we provide a scenario to give an example of how such an emergency might arise in the dental surgery. We also discuss the causes, signs and symptoms, prevention and management of the condition as well as providing additional background information where appropriate.

ACUTE CHEST PAIN

CLINICAL SCENARIO

George Richardson is a 62-year-old retired builder. He retired several years ago on medical grounds because of chest pains brought on by exertion. He has a fear of surgery, including dental surgery, and has therefore turned down the opportunity to have a coronary artery bypass graft to treat his angina on several occasions. He is booked in to have a broken down molar extracted. It is a straight forward extraction under local anaesthetic. However, he is clearly anxious as you prepare the local anaesthetic and starts to complain of chest pains. He is suffering an angina attack. What would you do next?

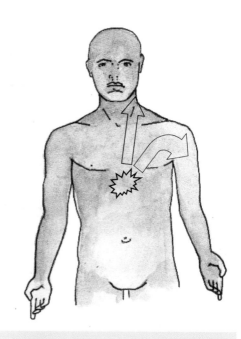

Figure 4.1. Chest pain of angina and acute MI radiates to left arm and neck

CAUSES

Severe acute chest pain is usually the result of myocardial ischaemia. The main differential diagnosis is between angina (reversible ischaemia) and myocardial infarction (irreversible ischaemia). Either may be precipitated by exercise, stress, emotion or anxiety.

SIGNS AND SYMPTOMS

- Severe, crushing retrosternal pain
- Pain may radiate to the arm neck and jaw, usually on the left side

Features suggesting angina

- The pain is short lasting and is relieved by rest and glyceryl trinitrate (GTN)

Features suggesting myocardial infarction (MI)

- The pain of MI is persistent and more severe
- The pain is not eased by rest or GTN
- In addition there may be breathlessness, nausea and vomiting, loss of consciousness and the pulse may be weak or irregular

---

PREVENTION

- Take a good medical history
- Identify patients with a history of angina, myocardial infarct or other cardiovascular disease
- As far as possible, keep to appointment times for such patients

Do not overburden their capacity for exertion

- If possible, use a downstairs surgery
- Ensure they have taken their normal medication
- If they are supposed to carry any drugs for prophylaxis of angina, such as glyceryl trinitrate, ensure they are readily to hand while they are in the dental surgery
- It is essential to minimise stress, anxiety and pain in patients with a history of angina.

MANAGEMENT

- If the patient has their own anti-angina drugs, these should be administered, otherwise use glyceryl trinitrate spray sublingually

- Monitor carefully until the angina pain has resolved

- Postpone planned treatment until another occasion

If there is no relief of pain in 3 minutes, the cause is likely to be an infarct

- Summon assistance - call for an ambulance

- Keep the patient sitting up - laying them flat may make breathlessness worse

- If you have an RA machine, give nitrous oxide and oxygen (50/50) to relieve pain and anxiety

- If nitrous oxide is not available, give oxygen

- If the patient is not allergic, give 150mg aspirin (1/2 a 300mg tablet). This can be left to dissolve in the buccal sulcus or swallowed if the patient is able

- Reassure the patient

If the patient loses consciousness, initiate **basic/advanced life support** as described in Section 2

BACKGROUND INFORMATION[48-52]

The early management of an acute myocardial infarction in a hospital setting has rapidly developed in the last 20 years. The benefits of achieving early patency of the affected coronary arteries are well recognised and this is the basis of thrombolytic therapy. Once a diagnosis of acute myocardial infarction has been confirmed in hospital, thrombolytic agents such as streptokinase can be given intravenously to break the causative thrombus down. Studies show that mortality can be halved if thrombolytic treatment is received within an hour of the onset of a myocardial infarct, with the benefit diminishing thereafter. Over 70% of eligible patients now receive thrombolysis within 30 minutes of arrival in hospital in the U.K. In an attempt to reduce the delay to thrombolysis even further, trials have been taking place to look at the feasibility of paramedics giving thrombolytic agents before the patient reaches hospital. This appears to reduce the mortality rate with no important associated hazards.

Primary angioplasty is another way of restoring coronary blood flow quickly after acute myocardial infarction and may be more effective than thrombolytic treatment, as it achieves higher coronary arterial patency rates and improved coronary flow. Primary angioplasty is a procedure in which a catheter is introduced into the coronary arteries and a balloon is inflated in the artery around the blockage to reopen the occluded section of artery. Ideally it would be carried out as soon as possible after diagnosis but limited resources often prevent this from happening. The advantages of thrombolysis and primary angioplasty may be complimentary and, should this be the case, will radically alter acute management of myocardial infarction in the future.

Pre-hospital thrombolysis is likely to become more common in rural areas and congested urban areas where transfer to hospital is likely to be delayed. Thus summoning an ambulance as soon as possible for a patient who is thought to be suffering a myocardial infection remains very important.

ACUTE ASTHMATIC ATTACK

CLINICAL SCENARIO

Cara Sylvester is a 20-year-old bank clerk. She is a regular attender at your practice and you have been treating her since she was a child. You remember that she used to have bad hayfever and asthma when younger for which she was always on medication. She has telephoned the practice today to say that she has toothache and you agree to see her. She is late for the appointment and has had to run to get there on time. On entering the surgery she is out of breath. She tells you about the toothache, mentioning that she has just taken some aspirin for the pain. Her breathlessness does not improve and she has an audible wheeze. She sits in the dental chair but her breathlessness gets worse and she insists on getting up. Standing up, she leans on the arm of the chair with her chest heaving for breath. She is having an acute asthma attack. What do you do next?

CAUSES

Exposure to an allergen, anxiety, cold, exercise or infection can precipitate an acute asthmatic attack in a patient predisposed to bronchospasm. Most attacks come on rapidly (within 30 minutes) and occur in patients with a known history. An acute asthma attack should not be taken lightly; if a patient fails to respond rapidly to treatment, they should be referred to hospital.

SIGNS AND SYMPTOMS

- Breathlessness and a tight chest
- Wheezing on expiration
- Accessory muscles of respiration in action

If the patient is unable to speak, you are dealing with a potentially fatal episode

---

PREVENTION

Avoid anxiety, pain and known allergens.

Ensure that the patient has had their normal prophylactic medication and has their bronchodilator readily available.

If a nebuliser is not available a similar effect can be obtained by administering two puffs of a bronchodilator into a large volume spacer and getting the patient to inhale through the spacer (see Section 1). This can be repeated every few seconds up to a maximum of 20 times (40 puffs). A makeshift large volume spacer can be formed by administering the bronchodilator through a hole in the base of a large disposable cup or 500ml soft drink bottle that the patient holds to their mouth.

MANAGEMENT

- Keep the patient sitting upright - laying them flat will increase breathlessness
- Encourage them to use the bronchodilator they normally use
- Offer a salbutamol inhaler if they do not have their own available
- If available administer nebulised salbutamol 5mg (Ventolin®) or terbutaline 10mg (Bricanyl®) with oxygen
- Give oxygen

Note: bronchodilator inhalers are blue, steroid inhalers are brown.

If the patient continues to be distressed

- Call for an ambulance
- Give 200mg hydrocortisone i/v (or i/m)

If the patient is unable or too distressed to use an inhaler or nebuliser, give

- Salbutamol 500 micrograms i/m

or

- Epinephrine (adrenaline) 0.5mL of 1:1,000 solution i/m if asthma is part of an anaphylactic reaction

---

BACKGROUND INFORMATION[53-56]

The reported incidence of asthma is increasing both in Britain and worldwide. Most people with asthma are atopic and have a tendency to suffer with eczema, hayfever, rhinitis, and other allergies. Contact with a sensitiser causes inflammation and narrowing of the airways resulting in the asthma symptoms of difficulty in breathing (mainly on expiration), wheezing, chest tightness, and cough. Such effects can be measured with a peak flow meter.

Acute asthmatic attacks can be stimulated by environmental allergens, exercise and respiratory viral infections. Attacks can be fatal and should be treated promptly. If, during an attack, a patient cannot complete a sentence in one breath, has a pulse rate greater than 110 beats per minute, has a respiratory rate greater than 25 breaths per minute or a peak flow rate less than 50% of best, then transfer to hospital is warranted. In general less than 20% of people presenting to an emergency department with asthma are actually admitted to hospital and of these, fewer than 10% require mechanical ventilation.

A systematic review has indicated that delivering an inhaled bronchodilator via a spacer device can be as effective as using a nebuliser in the treatment of an acute asthmatic attack. In developing countries, commercially produced spacers are generally unavailable or too expensive. This has led to efficacy testing of home-made devices. A 500ml plastic soft-drink bottle with a hole cut in its base for the metered dose inhaler to be inserted, and the bottle opening used as a mouthpiece has been found to be as efficient as a conventional spacer. A polystyrene drinks cup converted for use as a spacer was found to be less efficient, although still able to produce clinically important improvement. All plastic spacers have an electrostatic surface charge that reduces their efficiency. This can be overcome by priming the spacer with several puffs of bronchodilator or rinsing in detergent before use.

INHALED FOREIGN BODY

CLINICAL SCENARIO

Carl Spitz is a 15-year-old patient whom you have referred for orthodontic treatment. At an appointment with the orthodontist for fitting of a fixed appliance, the orthodontist loses control of one of the premolar brackets. The bracket drops to the back of his throat and in the scramble to get hold of the bracket, the orthodontist causes him to retch and the bracket disappears from sight. Carl is encouraged to rinse his mouth out, but there is no sign of the bracket. The orthodontist explains to his mother and him what has happened and that it is likely that the bracket has been swallowed or inhaled. What should the orthodontist do next?

SIGNS AND SYMPTOMS

Upper airways obstruction

- An object lodged in the upper airway will stimulate a cough reflex
- If the patient is choking, the object is large enough to cause respiratory obstruction
- The patient may grasp their throat

If the object blocks the airway completely they will be silent, unable to breathe or speak

- The skin will become cyanosed; this is especially evident in the lips
- They will make exaggerated efforts to take breath
- Eventually they will lose consciousness

Lower airways obstruction

The patient may be totally unaware that they have inhaled anything

CAUSES

Inhalation of a foreign body such as a tooth, inlay, crown or reamer is an ever-present risk in dentistry. An object lodged in the upper airways may cause respiratory obstruction. Smaller objects may be inhaled into the lower airways where if left unattended they may result in a lung abscess.

PREVENTION

This event is far easier to prevent than to treat and the use of a rubber dam will prevent all but the most bizarre incidents. An efficient high volume aspirator is also useful in aiding retrieval of any object dropped in the mouth. Be especially careful when trying in crowns or inlays or using small instruments in the mouth, ensure that burs are properly secured in the handpiece.

MANAGEMENT 1

If the patient is not choking or having difficulty breathing

- Check if the object is still in their mouth or clothing

If the object cannot be found or is known to have fallen into the throat:

- If the patient is supine, do not allow them to sit up but place the dental chair head down, allowing gravity to return the object to the oropharynx from where it may be retrieved
- Rolling the patient into the recovery position and encouraging them to cough may also help

If the object cannot be retrieved:

- Explain to the patient what has happened
- Refer to a hospital accident and emergency department for further assessment (chest and abdominal radiographs may be taken – a further sample of the lost object shown to the accident and emergency doctor can help with assessment and radiographic identification)
- If the object is found to be in the gastrointestinal tract (i.e., to have been swallowed), it is normally left to pass *per rectum*
- If the object is found to be in the respiratory tract, removal may require endoscopy or thoracic surgery

MANAGEMENT 2

If the object is larger and is causing breathing difficulties or choking

- Encourage the patient to cough forcefully to dislodge the object
- Lean the patient forward and give up to 5 sharp blows between the shoulder blades (*Figure 4.2*)
- If this fails, give up to 5 abdominal thrusts (*Figure 4.3*)
- If this fails re-check the mouth and remove any obstruction and continue to alternate 5 back blows with 5 abdominal thrusts

DISLODGING AN OBJECT FROM THE AIRWAY

Back blows

Lean the patient forward so that when the obstructing object is dislodged it is ejected from the mouth rather than going further down the airway. A good way to do this is to lean the patient over a chair. Give up to 5 sharp blows between the shoulder blades with the heel of your hand.

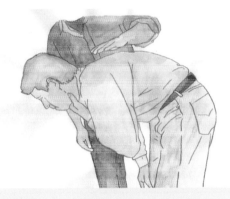

Figure 4.2. Back blows to dislodge an inhaled object

Abdominal thrusts (the Heimlich manoeuvre)

Form a fist with one hand and grip it with the other hand while encircling the patient with your arms from behind: your arms should be positioned just below the patient's ribs. Pull upwards and towards you, delivering a firm, upward inward thrust to the patient's diaphragm to expel air and the object from the chest.

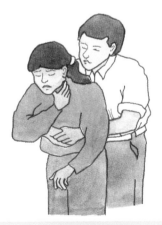

Figure 4.3. Abdominal thrusts (Heimlich manoeuvre)

At any time the patient may become unconscious. Unconsciousness may relax the muscles around the larynx and allow air to pass into the lungs.

MANAGEMENT 3

If the patient becomes <u>unconscious</u>

- Lay them flat
- Open the airway by tilting the head back and lifting the chin
- Check for breathing: **look, listen, feel**
- Attempt to give 2 'rescue breaths' by mouth to mouth ventilation

If effective breaths <u>can</u> be given:

- Check circulation
- If there is no circulation start basic life support (BLS)
- If circulation is present, continue mouth to mouth ventilation until the patient regains consciousness.
- Monitor circulation

If effective breaths <u>cannot</u> be given:

- Immediately start chest compressions. Do not wait to check circulation. The chest compressions may dislodge the object.
- After 15 compressions check mouth for obstruction and attempt rescue breaths again
- Repeat cycle of 15 compressions and 2 rescue breaths as necessary

BACKGROUND INFORMATION[57-59]

Judging by the paucity of discussion of this subject in the literature, this type of event, although common, probably only rarely causes serious problems. It is definitely an area where prevention is better than cure, so the use of a rubber dam or a gauze swab placed loosely over the back of the mouth and tethering of fine hand instruments is advisable. Take extra care with those patients who may have a reduced gag reflex, such as those under sedation, who are more at risk of swallowing or inhaling an object. Positioning of the patient may be a factor; some believe that treating patients while they are supine decreases the risk of aspiration or swallowing, while others believe that this increases the likelihood of these events occurring. There are reports of objects passing into the trachea without eliciting a cough or any other symptom suggesting inhalation.

The effect of a foreign object passing into the oropharynx depends on its size and shape and where it ends up. A sharp metallic object could theoretically pierce the lining mucosa at any point of its journey either into the respiratory or gastro-intestinal (GI) tracts and cause a mediastinal or abdominal infection. A pneumothorax may result if the lung wall is pierced. It may become impacted in the oropharynx; an object large enough to block the opening to the trachea may obstruct the airway and cause the patient to choke. If the object enters the respiratory tract it will lodge in the bronchial tree and it is important that it is retrieved as quickly as possible. The intense inflammatory response provoked by the object will make removal by brochoscopy much more difficult if there is delay and surgical removal may then become necessary.

If the object passes down the oesophagus into the stomach, more than likely it will pass uneventfully through the GI tract. Sharp objects, such as reamers, tend to pass through the intestines with the sharp end trailing in the centre of the faeces once they reach the transverse colon. Bloody stools or abdominal pain suggest perforation of the gut wall. Many authorities suggest chest and abdominal radiographs to locate the object and, if it is in the GI tract, serial radiographs to monitor its passage. However, in the absence of symptoms, some may think repeated irradiation of the abdomen and reproductive system, especially in growing patients, to be excessive.

Results from a British survey suggest that objects passing beyond reach into the oropharynx are approximately 30 times more likely to be swallowed than inhaled. According to a review of the Japanese literature, the majority of dental foreign objects swallowed or inhaled were

dentures and the majority of instruments 'lost' during dental treatment were reamers.

HYPERVENTILATION

CLINICAL SCENARIO
Kevin Peters is 23 and is not fond of the dentist; he attends only when he absolutely has to. He has been kept awake for a few days with toothache and its getting worse. Coupled with that, he now has a painful swelling of the left side of his jaw. He attends your surgery this morning; he is pale, sweaty and nervous. You examine him and explain that he has an abscess that needs attention. Then you give him an I.D. block as you intend to incise the abscess and drain the pus. After you give him the local anaesthetic he starts to breathe deeply and becomes pale. He is in a big panic and over-breathing. His panic is worsened when he notices that his hands have frozen in an odd position. What are you going to do next?

CAUSES
Extremely anxious or hysterical patients may hyperventilate in response to the stress of the dental surgery environment. This over-breathing washes out carbon dioxide from the lungs which results in over-excitability of nerves. They may complain of dizziness and tingling around the mouth; there may also be paraesthesia and tetany which is caused by hyper-excitability of nerves, characterised by spasms of skeletal muscle, especially the hands (carpo-pedal spasm) and the larynx. If severe, there may be laryngospasm, which can obstruct the airway, and cerebral vasoconstriction, which can eventually lead to collapse.

SIGNS AND SYMPTOMS
- Hyperventilation
- Flushed appearance
- Anxious or distressed
- Rapid pulse

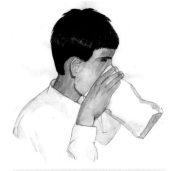

Figure 4.4. Patient re-breathing their expired air using a paper bag

MANAGEMENT
- Reassurance and explanation
- Get the patient to re-breathe their expired air by breathing in and out of a paper bag held over the mouth and nose (*Figure 4.4*)

PREVENTION
- Anxiety is the main precipitating factor for the hyperventilation response
- A calm, inviting reception and friendly staff
- Avoid keeping patients waiting and attend to their anxieties
- Reassurance and pain free dentistry are important preventative measures.
- In a patient with a previous history of hyperventilation, prophylaxis with an anxiolytic may be helpful e.g. temazepam 10mg the night before and 20mg one hour before surgery. If tachycardia is a particular problem, prescription of a beta blocker by the patient's GP may be helpful.

BACKGROUND INFORMATION[60]
When a patient hyperventilates, the excessive, hysterical over-breathing causes the patient to blow off carbon dioxide (CO_2). The partial pressure of CO_2 in the circulation falls (hypocapnia) and the blood pH rises (respiratory alkalaemia). There is a fall in the level of calcium ions and a consequent increase in nerve excitability. This causes numbness and tingling (paraesthesia) of the hands, feet and face and can be followed by muscle spasms of hands and feet (tetany) and stiffness of the face and lips, all of which may increase the anxiety. The alkalosis causes a constriction of cerebral blood flow resulting in blurred vision, dizziness and light-headedness. Loss of consciousness is not common as the cerebral hypoxia, resulting from vasoconstriction, causes the vessel walls to relax and the cerebral blood flow is re-established.

The episode of hyperventilation and the resulting alkalosis reduces the respiratory drive due to carbon dioxide and may well be followed by a period of depressed or even absent breathing then a period of intermittent breathing. This results in a build up of carbon dioxide in the blood and reversal of the alkalosis so that normal breathing eventually resumes. Increasing the CO_2 concentration of the inhaled air, by getting the patient to re-breath their expired air, reverses the physiological changes induced by hyperventilation.

ANGIO-OEDEMA

CLINICAL SCENARIO

Victor Goldbloom is a 45-year-old car sales executive. He is a regular patient of yours and you have treated him before on several occasions without any problems. His family doctor has recently put him on an exercise regime and an ACE inhibitor as he was found to be overweight and moderately hypertensive at his last check up. You have three composite restorations to do at this visit. The treatment goes well but when you remove the rubber dam, you notice that Mr Goldbloom's lips are noticeably swollen. He has angio-oedema of the lips. What do you do next?

Angio-oedema is a rare condition characterised by the sudden onset of localised swelling which usually fades over the subsequent 24-48 hours. The face, mouth and throat are commonly involved. Severe swelling of the upper respiratory tract may lead to respiratory obstruction and can be fatal.

CAUSES

Non-allergic angio-oedema may be hereditary or acquired. Hereditary angio-oedema is due to an inherited defect in the production or function of C^1 esterase inhibitor, a component of the complement cascade. The consequence is an overactive or sensitive complement system which, when triggered, results in uncontrolled tissue oedema. Acquired angio-oedema is usually idiopathic in origin although several predisposing factors have been identified including drugs, such as angiotensin converting enzyme (ACE) inhibitors and analgesics. In a susceptible individual an acute attack may be precipitated by the simple manipulation of the oral tissues that normally occurs during dental treatment.

The term 'allergic angio-oedema' is used to describe a type 1 allergic response with tissue swelling affecting the face, mouth

---

SIGNS AND SYMPTOMS
- Oedematous facial swelling of rapid onset
- Swelling of tongue or soft palate
- Respiratory difficulty

and throat. If severe it may be accompanied by profound hypotension causing the patient to lose consciousness and collapse, in which case it is called anaphylaxis (see section on anaphylaxis). Allergic angio-oedema can be precipitated by allergens commonly used in dentistry such as latex or penicillin.

PREVENTION

Check medical history for previous episodes or family history. If the history is suggestive of angio-oedema, arrange for hospital investigation of the cause. Cases of hereditary angio-oedema should have any extractions or surgical procedures carried out in hospital with appropriate C^1 esterase inhibitor concentrate cover. If angio-oedema is allergic in origin, avoid known allergens.

MANAGEMENT

Depends on the severity of the reaction

Mild reaction: (mild tissue swelling, no respiratory difficulty, patient conscious)
- Give an oral antihistamine, e.g. chlorphenamine (chlorpheniramine) (Piriton®) 4mg four times daily for 5 days
- Arrange a review and refer to hospital as appropriate

Moderate reaction: (more severe swelling with little or no respiratory difficulty and the patient is conscious)
- Give oxygen
- 10mg chlorphenamine (Piriton®) i/m or slowly i/v
- 200mg hydrocortisone i/m or i/v
- Call an ambulance

Severe reaction: (severe tissue swelling/ respiratory difficulty or patient unconscious)
- Treat as anaphylaxis

BACKGOUND INFORMATION[61-62]

Angio-oedema describes oedema in the subcutaneous tissues which occurs quickly and then gradually subsides over a day or two. Urticaria (a blotchy rash, usually white or pink on reddened skin) can also occur in association with the angio-oedema. Although allergy is sometimes the cause, many patients develop these problems for non-allergic reasons. When true allergy is the cause, the relationship between exposure to the substance causing the allergic reaction and the development of the reaction itself is usually clear. In idiopathic angiodema and urticaria, the rash and swellings often occur with no pattern or relationship to any trigger factor. In these cases the mast cells become hyper-responsive and release histamine in response to simple stimuli such as pressure (including manipulation of the oral tissues), heat or cold or for no obvious reason. Factors that can increase the hyper-responsiveness of mast cells include drugs such as angiotensin converting enzyme (ACE) inhibitors and non-steroidal anti-inflammatory drugs (NSAIDS), some food colourings and preservatives, and following viral infection.

Angio-oedema secondary to ACE inhibitors has increased in frequency as these drugs have become more widely used in the treatment of cardiovascular disease. There seems to be some predilection for the resulting angio-oedema to affect the head and neck particularly, and deaths due to ACE inhibitor related angio-oedema have been recorded. There is evidence that people of Afro-Caribbean origin are more at risk than other racial groups. Awareness and identification of these groups of patients is important as alternative cardiovascular drugs are available.

Hereditary angio-oedema is a very rare cause of oedema which is due to an absolute or functional deficiency of C^1 esterase inhibitor. Patients suffering with this condition require specialised hospital management for oral surgery procedures.

VOMITING

CLINICAL SCENARIO

You have just completed a bridge preparation on you first patient of the afternoon and are ready to take the impressions. As you position the upper impression tray Mrs Brown starts to wretch and is clearly distressed by the procedure. Even though you remove the impression tray, she continues to retch, turns pale and starts to sweat profusely and then vomits. What would you do?

CAUSES

Much dentistry is carried out with the patient lying supine and there is the potential for patients to vomit while in this position, especially during impression taking. It may also occur during conscious sedation. There is also a chance that a patient who has just fainted and is unconscious may vomit and aspirate the vomit into the lungs, which is a potentially serious problem.

SIGNS AND SYMPTOMS

Vomiting is often preceded by:

- Feeling unwell or sick
- Pallor
- Sweating
- Salivation
- Retching

PREVENTION

Vomiting is more likely on a full stomach. Aspiration of vomit is the most serious consequence and this is more likely if the patient is supine, sedated or unconscious.

MANAGEMENT

If the patient is <u>conscious</u>

- Remove any instruments or loose items from the mouth
- Allow the patient to sit leaning forward
- Provide a receptacle for the vomit
- Reassure
- Provide good ventilation

If the patient is <u>unconscious</u>

- Put the patient into the recovery position
- Use suction to keep the mouth and airway clear

BACKGROUND INFORMATION

Vomiting is a primitive protective response. It is controlled by the vomiting centre in the medulla of the brain. This centre is close to those that control respiration and cardiac function. As such, the vomiting centre is not easily depressed by general anaesthesia unless it is so deep as to suppress the other vital centres, hence the risk of vomiting under general anaesthesia. Chemicals and bacterial toxins can induce vomiting and do so by stimulating chemosensitive receptors in the medulla close to the vomiting centre. Some general anaesthetic agents tend to stimulate these centres. Other receptors will also trigger vomiting, for example stretch or touch receptors in the pillars of the fauces. Vomiting can also be provoked by pain or emotional distress.

PANIC ATTACKS

CLINICAL SCENARIO
Zarina Patel is a very anxious 19-year-old who has been persuaded by her parents to visit your practice because she is experiencing pain from an impacted wisdom tooth. Her parents have warned you of her anxiety and your nurse and her mother gently persuade her into the surgery. However, on seeing the dental chair and equipment she starts to panic. She becomes very agitated, starts shaking, sweating profusely and becomes flushed. She complains that her mouth is very dry and her heart is about to explode. She is having a panic attack. What would you do next?

CAUSES

Panic attacks are discrete, recurrent attacks of acute anxiety. They begin suddenly and last usually about 10-30 minutes. They usually represent a morbid fear or anxiety out of all proportion to the situation. Most such phobias are centred on particular situations e.g. flying, general anaesthesia or dental treatment and patients generally protect themselves from attacks by avoiding the situations that precipitate them. Sometimes phobias can be part of a more severe disorder such as depression, personality disorder, obsessive neurosis or chronic anxiety state.

PREVENTION

Patients with phobias relating to dental treatment require careful, sympathetic handling and lots of patience. Often the anxiety is increased by a feeling that they have no control over the situation. A clear understanding of precisely what induces the phobia may allow the patient to undergo treatment by providing them with some control over the precipitating situation. Sometimes the use of anxiolytic drugs or conscious sedation will help patients undergo treatment.

Note: Hyperventilation is often a feature of a panic attack and should be treated by getting the patient to re-breath their expired air by holding a paper bag over their mouth and nose. See the section on hyperventilation.

SIGNS AND SYMPTOMS
- Sudden onset extreme anxiety or fear
- Palpitations
- Giddiness
- Tremor
- Sweating
- Flushing
- Shortness of breath or hyperventilation
- Paraesthesia
- Dry mouth
- Blurred vision
- Weakness

MANAGEMENT
- Recognise a panic attack for what it is - an anxiety condition rather than a serious medical problem
- Be sympathetic, reassuring and patient
- You may need to postpone treatment and withdraw the patient from the anxiety provoking situation
- Monitor the patient's recovery
- Consider carrying out further treatment with some form of anxiolytic regimen, such as Temazepam 10mg the night before and 20mg 1 hour before treatment

---

BACKGROUND INFORMATION

Panic attacks are sudden onset attacks of anxiety, out of all proportion to the cause, that are precipitated by a particular situation. They are usually accompanied by an alarming array of autonomically mediated symptoms that often increase the patient's level of anxiety. Sympathetic effects include palpitations (racing heart), chest tightness or pain, shortness of breath and hyperventilation, which may induce dizziness and paraesthesia. Parasympathetic effects may include nausea, an urge to defecate, blurred vision and weakness.

Attacks are frequently accompanied by a gross misinterpretation of the danger they represent. Patients fear dying, going mad or collapsing; they may be convinced that something terrible is happening to them - the sympathetic effects may lead them to believe they are having a heart attack. Attacks may be triggered by anxious thoughts or the anticipation of a phobic situation, such as a trip to the dentist.

AGGRESSIVE OR HOSTILE BEHAVIOUR

CLINICAL SCENARIO

George Bailey is a betting office clerk and an infrequent attender at your practice. Your receptionist and nursing staff don't like him as he often complains and is unpleasant to them, although you have never had any real problems with him yourself. As you are checking his notes before calling him into your surgery you hear raised voices in the waiting room. Soon after, you receptionist enters the room to warn you that Mr Bailey is complaining about being kept waiting and smells strongly of alcohol. Almost immediately he enters the room pushing the receptionist out of the way and accuses you of discussing him behind his back. He is clearly very agitated and aggressive. What do you do next?

CAUSES

Acute anxiety, often exacerbated by fear or pain, can cause perfectly normal individuals to become complaining, aggressive or panicky in the dental surgery. Hyperventilation may be a feature of anxiety or a hysterical personality (see sections on hyperventilation and panic attacks). Alcohol, drug abuse or organic disease such as diabetes, psychiatric disease or head injury may also result in abnormal behaviour.

Alcohol or drugs are often taken by patients in an attempt to relieve dental pain or to find the courage to attend the dentist. Diabetics who become hypoglycaemic may become irritable and aggressive, while patients with head injuries may show disturbed behaviour because of brain damage. Psychoses and psychiatric personality disorders may also result in abnormal behaviour.

SIGNS AND SYMPTOMS
- Anxiety
- Confusion
- Aggression
- Disturbed or difficult behaviour

PREVENTION

- A calm inviting reception with alert but friendly staff
- Sit down rather than stand to confront an aggressive individual
- Avoid keeping patients waiting and be aware of their anxieties
- Be alert to the patient's behaviour to anticipate any difficulties at an early stage
- Tact and diplomacy are probably paramount in preventing any problems
- If anxiety is the main problem, prophylaxis with an anxiolytic may be helpful e.g. temazepam 10mg the night before and 20mg 1 hour before surgery

---

MANAGEMENT

- Adopt a calm, understanding, and non-confrontational but firm approach
- Sit down rather than stand to confront them
- If the patient is unresponsive or difficult to manage, it is advisable to try and get them to return on another occasion
- If the patient becomes very aggressive or disturbed, call the police
- Do not put yourself or any members of staff at risk of injury from aggressive patients or their escorts

---

BACKGROUND INFORMATION[63-65]

Unfortunately, aggressive and hostile behaviour by patients towards healthcare workers is becoming an increasingly common occurrence. It has long been a problem in the emergency departments of hospitals, where the effects of alcohol and fear play a large part in the problem. However, in recent years there has been an increasing problem with violent and aggressive attacks on general medical practitioners and their staff. Although this probably occurs less frequently in dental practices, a survey of 3,078 dental practice staff (dentists and other staff) found that many had experienced some form of aggression at work. In general, practice staff were twice as likely to be the target of aggressive behaviour than dentists. The survey also recorded 25 incidents of physical assault by patients or their relatives. In this case dentists were twice as likely as staff to be the target.

ADVERSE REACTIONS TO LOCAL ANAESTHETIC INJECTIONS

CLINICAL SCENARIO

Sharon Woodward is booked in for removal of a lower left wisdom tooth. You are concerned it could turn into a surgical and decide to give plenty of local anaesthetic just in case. Soon after you have given the local anaesthetic you check to see if she has gone numb. She complains that she can't move the muscles on that side of her face. When you check, you notice that the skin over her left cheek and extending towards the temple has become blanched and she can't close her left eye or move the muscles on that side of her face. What do you do next?

CAUSES

The most common adverse reaction to injection of a local anaesthetic is a simple faint. Other causes of collapse following an injection, such as anaphylaxis, are very rare. Most other types of reaction associated with local anaesthetic injections are the result of intravascular injection, inaccurate placement or overdose.

PROBLEMS ASSOCIATED WITH LOCAL ANAESTHETIC INJECTIONS
- Faint
- Intravascular injection
- Injection into a muscle
- Facial palsy
- Cardiovascular reactions
- Local anaesthetic overdose
- Fractured needle
- Local anaesthetic allergy

INTRAVASCULAR INJECTION

CAUSES

Failure to aspirate correctly to check that the needle tip is not in a vessel before injecting or too rapid an injection.

SIGNS AND SYMPTOMS
Possible effects may include:
- Agitation
- Palpitations
- Confusion/drowsiness
- Failure of anaesthesia
- Fits or a loss of consciousness

PREVENTION

Use an aspirating syringe, aspirate correctly and inject slowly.

MANAGEMENT
- Lay the patient flat
- Maintain the airway
- Give oxygen
- Give reassurance

Most patients will recover spontaneously within half an hour. If fits or loss of consciousness supervene, institute appropriate management.

INJECTION INTO A MUSCLE

This occurs most commonly while attempting to give an inferior dental nerve block. It usually results in discomfort and trismus due to stretching or tearing of muscle fibres and haemorrhage into the muscle. The patient should be reassured and the situation explained. The pain and trismus will usually resolve over a few days. Gentle jaw exercises may speed this process and analgesics may help by reducing the pain. Since injection into a muscle is usually the result of a misplaced injection it is also often accompanied by failure of anaesthesia.

FACIAL PALSY

Temporary facial palsy, diplopia (double vision) or localised facial pallor occasionally occur when the local anaesthetic is misplaced or tracks towards the facial nerve or orbital contents. The patient should be reassured and if the eyelids are affected they should be closed and covered with a protective dressing until the anaesthetic wears off.

CARDIOVASCULAR REACTIONS

Palpitations are the most common cardiovascular reaction to the injection of local anaesthetic and is usually caused by the vasoconstrictor. Reactions occur most commonly following overdosage or intravascular injection. The patient should be reassured while the symptoms subside. If the reaction is severe, then treat as for chest pains.

LOCAL ANAESTHETIC OVERDOSE

Overdose with local anaesthetics is uncommon. The amount required to produce an overdose remains controversial; however, for a healthy adult an upper limit of 5 dental cartridges has been suggested. In children, the elderly and those with liver disease the upper limit will be considerably less. Overdose reactions vary from drowsiness to convulsions. You should reassure the patient, keep the airway patent and give oxygen. Rarely, respiratory failure or even cardiac arrest occur and should be treated appropriately.

NEEDLE FRACTURE

Modern disposable needles rarely fracture unless the needle is re-used or is repeatedly bent and straightened. If the protruding end of the broken needle cannot be grasped easily with mosquito forceps, the patient should be immediately referred to a surgeon for its removal.

LOCAL ANAESTHETIC ALLERGY

Allergy to local anaesthesia is very rare. Collapse following a local anaesthetic is far more likely to be due to a faint or another cause. If the allergic reaction is severe and life threatening, it is managed as for anaphylaxis. If the systemic reaction is less severe, without marked respiratory difficulty or symptomatic hypotension, then it should be managed as described for angio-oedema. See sections on anaphylaxis and angio-oedema for signs and symptoms and management.

POSTOPERATIVE BLEEDING

CLINICAL SCENARIO

Just before lunch you completed a relatively straightforward lower first molar extraction on Mr Wood. You return from lunch to find a lot of commotion in the waiting room. He is sitting with his hands full of bloody tissues that he is dabbing at his blood filled mouth. His wife is with him and very upset. What would you do next?

CAUSES

Post-extraction bleeding normally has a local cause, either gingival bleeding due to trauma to the soft tissues or oozing from damaged vessels in the socket. Anticoagulants and drugs that alter platelet function (e.g. aspirin) also predispose to haemorrhage. Systemic causes of bleeding are uncommon and can usually be identified by taking a careful medical history.

Primary haemorrhage occurs at the time of surgery and is caused by damage to the tissues. Reactionary haemorrhage usually occurs a few hours after surgery and is due to the effects of the vasoconstrictor in the local anaesthetic wearing off. Following an extraction it may also be the result of the blood clot being dislodged from the socket. Secondary haemorrhage occurs a few days after the procedure and is usually caused by post-operative wound infection. It is relatively uncommon following routine extractions.

PREVENTION

Take a careful medical history to identify any underlying medical condition or anticoagulant medication that could increase the risk of postoperative bleeding. Patients with a medical condition predisposing to haemorrhage should be referred to a hospital oral surgery unit for assessment and management of their extractions.

Patients on long acting anticoagulants e.g. warfarin, nicoumalone or phenindione should have their INR checked (most patients' INR is maintained between 2 and 4). If the INR is below 3 you can proceed with minor surgery

---

SIGNS AND SYMPTOMS
- Post extraction bleeding is usually quite obvious and may be alarming to the patient and their relatives. A little blood makes a lot of mess, particularly when mixed with saliva.

- To identify if bleeding is coming primarily from the soft tissue or the socket, pinch the soft tissues against the walls of the socket between forefinger and thumb. This usually stops soft tissue bleeding, while bleeding from the socket will continue to well up from within the socket.

MEDICAL CONDITIONS ASSOCIATED WITH INCREASED RISK OF HAEMORRHAGE
- Haemophilia A and B
- Von Willebrand's disease
- Vitamin K deficiency
- Liver disease
- Disseminated intravascular coagulation
- Fibrinolytic states and fibrinolytic drug therapy
- Other situations where coagulation may be affected include:
  Polycythaemia, myelofibrosis, leukaemia, lymphoma, chronic renal failure, gram-negative shock, following massive transfusions and where antibodies have developed to clotting factors

(simple extraction of up to 3 teeth, gingival surgery or single surgical tooth extraction) without anticoagulant dose adjustment. Any postoperative bleeding should be controlled by local measures. The socket should be packed with a resorbable haemostatic dressing and sutured (see below). If the anticoagulant dose requires adjustment this must be done in consultation with the patient's anticoagulant clinic. Do not instruct the patient to make these adjustments yourself. The INR should be checked within the 24 hours prior to the extractions. If possible a single extraction should be done first to confirm adequate haemostasis. More major surgery or patients with complicating medical history should be treated in hospital.

The risk of post extraction bleeding will be reduced by:
- Minimising trauma to the tissues at the time of surgery.
- Ensuring haemostasis before discharging the patient from the surgery.
- Providing postoperative instructions including advice on how to avoid dislodging the blood clot from the socket.

BACKGROUND INFORMATION[66-67]
Management of patients taking anticoagulant drugs is still an area of debate. Until recently, the general advice was that the INR should be adjusted to below 2-2.5 before extractions or other minor oral surgical procedures are

---

MANAGEMENT
- Reassure the patient and ask relatives to leave unless the patient is very young
- Clean the mouth with a swab soaked in saline and use suction to locate the source of bleeding
- Get the patient to bite firmly on a gauze swab, correctly located such that pressure is exerted over the socket, for ten minutes
- Enquire again into the patient's medical history, especially family history, drug history and previous operative history, to exclude systemic causes

If bleeding continues:
- Give local anaesthesia. This will often slow or stop the bleeding.

If bleeding is primarily from the gingival soft tissues:
- Use a horizontal mattress suture to compress the soft tissue vessels against the socket walls
- Apply local pressure by getting the patient to bite on a gauze swab
- Keep the patient rested until the bleeding stops

If bleeding is primarily from the socket:
- Insert an oxidised cellulose gauze or sponge (e.g. Surgicell®, Oxycell®) or a collagen sponge (e.g. Haemocollagen)
- Pack the socket (if available, use ribbon gauze soaked in Whitehead's varnish)
- Insert a horizontal mattress suture to compress the soft tissues and hold the pack in place
- Apply local pressure by getting the patient to bite on a gauze swab

Keep the patient rested until the bleeding stops

If it is not possible to identify if bleeding is from the soft tissues or socket:

Employ both the above approaches

If bleeding persists or if the patient is severely anaemic or debilitated, then admit to hospital

If the bleeding is uncontrollable, call an ambulance

performed. However, this advice has recently changed as a result of concern about the increased risk of thrombosis in patients whose INR is lowered prior to dental procedures. Current evidence suggests that this risk outweighs the increased risk of haemorrhage for patients undergoing dental procedures when the INR is below 3. Therefore, patients whose INR is 3 or under should not have their anticoagulant dose adjusted before undergoing simple minor oral surgical procedures. Post-operative bleeding should be prevented by the pre-emptive insertion of a haemostatic dressing into the socket, and suturing before getting the patient to bite firmly on a gauze pack placed over the socket. Current evidence suggests that local measures are effective in preventing post-operative haemorrhage in these patients and that other measures, such as the use of tranexamic acid provide no additional benefit in the general practice setting.

It is important to check if patients on anti-coagulants require antibiotic cover. Some cardiac conditions that require antibiotic cover are also treated with anti-coagulants e.g. patients with artificial heart valves. Current evidence suggests that it is safe to give a single dose of amoxicillin or clindamycin for this purpose, although occasionally changes in INR have been reported following their use. Many drugs have the potential to interact with anticoagulants; for example aspirin and other non-steroidal anti-inflammatory drugs (NSAIDs), carbamazepine, antibiotics such as metronidazole, and antifungals. When prescribing drugs for a patient who is taking warfarin, the potential for interaction should always be considered and checked in a suitable reference source such as the BNF. If analgesics are required, paracetamol should be used.

Many patients now take antiplatelet medication to prevent cardiovascular disease or stroke. These drugs include:

- Low dose aspirin (75-300mg daily)
- Clopidogrel
- Dipyridamole.

Current evidence suggests that this therapy should not be stopped or altered prior to dental surgical procedures in primary care. Their effect on primary haemostasis is minimal and easily controlled by normal local measures.

Appendix

1. BDA 64 Wimpole Street, London, W1G 8YS. Tel: 020 7935 0875. Email: enquires@bda.org Web: www.bda-dentistry.org.uk

2. Admor Limited, Kings Close, Yapton, West Sussex BN18 0EX. Tel: 01243 553078. Fax: 01243 555017. Email: print@admor.co.uk Web: www.admor.co.uk

3. Scully C, Cawson RA. *Medical Problems in Dentistry.* 5th ed. Edinburgh: Elsevier, 2005.

4. Vitalograph Ltd, Maids Moreton, Buckingham, MK18 1SW. Tel: 01280 827110. Fax: 01280 823302. Web: www.vitalograph.co.uk

5. Crestline Coach Ltd., 802 - 57th St E, Saskatoon, SK, S7K 5Z1, Canada. Email: info@crestlinecoach.com Web: www.crestlinecoach.com

6. Laerdal Medical Ltd., Laerdal House, Goodmead Road, Orpington, Kent, BR6 0HX. Tel: 01689 876634. Fax: 01689 873800). Email: customer.service@laerdal.co.uk Web: www.laerdal.co.uk

7. AMBU products available from Keith McCallum, Medicotest UK Ltd., Burrel Road, St Ives, Cambs, PE27 3LE. Tel: 01480 498403. Fax: 01480 498405. Email kmccallum@medicotest.co.uk Web: www.ambu.com

8. Portex Safe Response mouth to mask adult resuscitator. Portex Ltd, Boundary Road, Hythe, Kent CT21 6JL. Tel: 01303 260551. Fax: 01303 266761. Email: info@portex.com Web: www.portex.com

9. Timesco Rescu-mask. Timesco of London, Timesco House, 1 Knights Road, London E16 2AT. Tel: 020 7511 9960. Fax: 020 7511 7888. Email: info@timesco.com Web: www.timesco.com

10. Blackwells, Medcare House, Centurion Close, Gillingham Business Park, Gillingham, Kent ME8 0SB. Tel: 01634 877620. Fax: 01634 877621.

11. BOC Customer Service Centre, Priestley Road, Worsley, Manchetser, M28 2UT. Tel: 0800 111333. Fax: 0800 111555. Web: www.bocmedical.co.uk

12. Linde Gas UK Ltd, Johnsons Bridge Road, Church Lane, West Bromwich, B71 1LG. Tel: 0121 500 1000. Fax: 0121 500 1111. Web: www.linde-gas.co.uk

13. Life Tec Medical Ltd, Crown Industrial Estate, Canal Road, Timperley, Altrincham, Cheshire, WA14 1TF. Tel: 0161 926 0000. Fax: 0161 926 0002. Email: info@lifetechmedical.com Web: www.lifetecmedical.com

14. Medtronic Limited, Suite One, Sherbourne House, Croxley Business Park, Watford, WD18 8WW. Tel: 01923 212213. Fax: 01923 241004. Web: www.medtronic-ers.com

15. Philips Medical Systems, The Observatory, Castlefield Road, Reigate Surrey, RH2 0FV. Tel: 0870 607 7677. Fax: 0870 607 7688. Email: CMS.enquiries@Philips.com Web: www.medical.philips.com

16. National Dental Advisory Committee. Emergency dental drugs. Edinburgh: The Scottish Office, Department of Health, February 1999.

17. Scully C, Cawson R A. *Medical Problems in Dentistry.* 5th ed. p564. Edinburgh: Elsevier, 2005.

18. Crosby A C. Medical Emergencies. In Figures KH and Lamb DJ (eds) *Primary and emergency dental care: a practitioner's guide.* pp 156-164. Oxford: Wright, 1995.

19. Malamed S F. *Medical emergencies in the dental office* 5th ed. p65. St Louis: Mosby, 2000.

20. Gill D S, Sharma V, Whitbread M. Emergency drugs in dental practice. *Dent Update* 1998; **25:** 450-460.

21. Girdler NM, Grieveson B. The emergency drug box - time for action? *Br Dent J* 1999; **187:** 77-78.

22. Min-i-jet system. UK Distribution: P and D Pharmaceuticals, 38 Woolmer Way, Bordon, Hants., GU35 9QF. Tel: 01420 487501. Fax: 01420 478315. Web: www.pdpharm.co.uk

23. Martindale Pharmaceuticals Ltd and Aurum Pharmaceuticals Ltd, Hubert Road, Brentwood, Essex, CM14 4LZ. Tel: 01277 266600. Fax: 01277 848976. Web: www.martindalepharma.co.uk

24. Resuscitation Council (UK), 5th Floor, Tavistock House North, Tavistock Square, London WC1H 9HR. Tel: 020 7388 4678. Fax: 020 7383 0773. Email: enquiries@resus.org Web: www.resus.org.uk

25. Speirs RL Some reflections on the mechanism of the common faint. *Dent Update* 1983; **10**: 644-650.

26. Salins PC, Kuriakose M, Sharma SM, Tauro, DP. Hypogylcemia as a possible factor in the induction of vaso-vagal syncope. *Oral Surg, Oral Med, Oral Path* 1992; **74**: 544-549.

27. Valenzuela TD, Roe DJ, Nichol G, Clark LL, Spaite DW, Hardman RG. Outcomes of rapid defibrillation by security officers after cardiac arrest in casinos. *N Engl J Med 2000;* **343**: 1206-1209.

28. Liddle R, Davies CS, Colquhoun M, Handly AJ. The automated external defibrillator. *BMJ 2003;* **327**: 1216-1218.

29. European Resuscitation Council Guidelines 2000 for automated defibrillation. *Resuscitation* 2001; **48**: 207-209.

30. Jowett NI, Cabot LB. Diabetic hypoglycaemia and the dental patient. *Br Dent J* 1998; **185**: 439-442.

31. The Diabetics Control and Complications Trial Research Group. The effect of intensive treatment of diabetics on the development and progression of long-term complications in insulin dependent diabetes mellitus. *N Engl J Med* 1993; **329**: 977-986.

32. Fagot-Campagna A, Narayan KM, Imperatore G. Type 2 diabetes in children. *BMJ* 2001; **322**: 377-378.

33. Nicholson G, Burrin JM, Hall GM. Perioperative steroid supplementation. *Anaesthesia* 1998; **53**: 1091-1104.

34. Thomason JM, Girdler NM, Kendall-Taylor P, Wastell H, Weddel A, Seymour RA. An investigation into the need for supplementary steroids in organ transplant patients undergoing gingival surgery. A double-blind, split-mouth, cross-over study. *J Clin Periodontol* 1999; **26**: 577-582.

35. Friedman RJ, Schiff CF, Bromberg JS. Use of supplementary steroids in patients having orthopaedic operations. *J Bone Joint Surg* 1995; **77**: 1801-1806.

36. Miller CS, Little JW, Falace DA. Supplementary corticosteroids for dental patients with adrenal insufficiency: reconsideration of the problem. *JADA* 2001; **132**: 1570-1579.

37. Project team of the Resuscitation Council (UK). The emergency medical treatment of anaphylactic reactions. *J Accid Emerg Med* 1999; **16**: 243-247.

38. Resuscitation Council (UK). Project Team report on the emergency medical treatment of anaphylactic reactions. Available at: www.resus.org.uk

39. Schierhout G, Roberts I. Fluid resuscitation with colloid or crystalloid solutions in critically ill patients: a systematic review of randomised trials. *BMJ* 1998; **316**: 961-964.

40. Turpeinen M, Kuokkanen J, Backman A. Adrenaline and nebulised salbutamol in acute asthma. *Arch Dis Child* 1984; **59**: 666-668.

41. Sheikh A, Alves B. Hospital admissions for acute anaphylaxis: time trend study. *BMJ* 2000; **320**: 1441.

42. Treatment of convulsive status epilepticus. Recommendations of the Epilepsy Foundation of America's Working Group on Status Epilepticus. *J Am Med Ass* 1993; **270**: 854-859.

43. Smith D, Defalla BA, Chadwick DW. The misdiagnosis of epilepsy and the management of refractory epilepsy in a specialist clinic. *QJM* 1999; **92**: 15-23.

44. Lowenstein DH, Allredge BK. Current concepts: status epilepticus. *N Engl J Med* 1998; **338**: 970-976.

45. Scott RC, Besag FM, Neville BG. Buccal midazolam and rectal diazepam for treatment of prolonged seizures in childhood and adolescence: a randomised trial. *Lancet* 1999; **353**: 623-626.

46. Bath PM, Lees KR. ABC of arterial and venous disease. Acute stroke. *BMJ* 2000; **320**: 920-923.

47. Hacke W, Brott T, Caplan L, Meier D *et al.* Thrombolysis in acute ischaemic stroke: controlled trials and clinical experience. *Neurology* 1999; **53**: S3-14.

48. Fibrinolytic Therapy Trialists (FTT) Collaborative Group. Indications for fibrinolytic therapy in suspected acute myocardial infarction: collaborative overview of early morbidity and major mortality results from all randomised trials of more than 1000 patients. *Lancet* 1994; **343**: 311-322.

49. Boersma E, Maas ACP, Dekkers JW, Simoons MI. Early thrombolytic treatment in acute myocardial infarction: reappraisal of the golden hour. *Lancet* 1996; **348:** 771-775.

50. Morrison LJ, Verbeek PR, McDonald AC, Sawadsky BV, Cook DJ. Mortality and pre-hospital thrombolysis for acute myocardial infarction: a meta-analysis. *J Am Med Ass* 2000; **283:** 2686-2692.

51. Keeley EC, Boura JA, Grines CL. Primary angioplasty versus intravenous thrombolytic therapy for acute myocardial infarction: a quantitative review of 23 randomised trials. *Lancet* 2003; **361:** 13-20.

52. Jowett NI, Cabot LB. Patients with cardiac disease: considerations for the dental practitioner. *Br Dent J* 2000; **189:** 297-302.

53. Kaur B, Anderson HR, Austin J et al. Prevalence of asthma symptoms, diagnosis, and treatment in 12-14 year old children across Great Britain (international study of asthma and allergies in childhood, ISAAC (UK). *BMJ* 1998; **316:** 118-124.

54. Cates C. Holding chamber versus nebulisers for β agonist treatment of acute asthma. *Cochrane Database Syst Rev* 2000.

55. Zar HJ, Brown G, Donson H, Braithwaite N, Mann MD, Weinberg EG. Home-made spacers for bronchodilator therapy in children with acute asthma: a randomised trial. *Lancet* 1999; **354:** 979-982.

56. Wildhaber JH, Devadason SG, Hayden MJ et al. Electrostatic charge on a plastic spacer device influences the delivery of salbutamol. *Eur Respir J* 1996; **9:** 1943-1946.

57. Atherton GJ, McCaul JA, Williams SA. Medical emergencies in general dental practice in Great Britain. Part 1: their prevalence over a 10-year period. *Br Dent J* 1999; **186:** 72-79.

58. Tamura N, Nakajima T, Matsumoto S, Ohyama T, Ohashi Y. Foreign bodies of dental origin in the air and food passages. *Int J Oral Maxillofac Surg* 1986; **15:** 739-751.

59. Resuscitation Council (UK). Guidelines for dealing with choking as part of Basic Life Support. Available at: www.resus.org.uk

60. Speirs RL, Barsby MJ. Hyperventilation in the dental chair. *Dent Update* 1995; **22:** 95-98.

61. Sabroe RA, Black AK. Angiotensin-converting enzyme (ACE) inhibitors and angio-oedema. *Br J Dermatol* 1997; **136:** 153-158.

62. Pavletic AJ. Late angio-oedema in patients taking angiotensin-converting-enzyme inhibitors. *Lancet* 2002; **360:** 493-494.

63. Pemberton MN, Atherton GJ, Thornhill MH. Violence and aggression at work. *Br Dent J* 2000; **189:** 409-410.

64. BDA advisory service. Violence at work (advice sheet D14). London: British Dental Association, 1997. www.bda-dentistry.org.uk

65. Survey into violence and abuse against dental practitioners and their staff. London: British Dental Association, 1997. www.bda-dentistry.org.uk

66. UK Medical Information Service, NHS Executive, North West Medical Information Centre. Surgical management of the primary care dental patient on warfarin, 2001. www.ukmi.nhs.uk

67. UK Medical Information Service, NHS Executive, North West Medical Information Centre. Surgical management of the primary care dental patient on antiplatelet medication, 2001. www.ukmi.nhs.uk